History and Physical for the Pediatric Dental Patient

S. Thikkurissy · Sara Golkari

Editors

History and Physical for the Pediatric Dental Patient

Establishing a Systematic Approach for Procedural Sedation

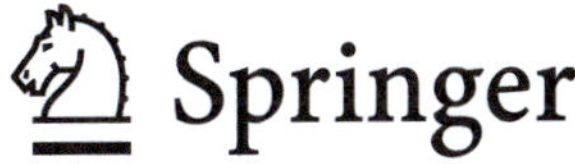 Springer

Editors
S. Thikkurissy
Division of Dentistry
Cincinnati Children's Hospital Medical
Cincinnati, OH, USA

Sara Golkari
Private Practice
Chicago, IL, USA

ISBN 978-3-031-51460-9   ISBN 978-3-031-51458-6   (eBook)
https://doi.org/10.1007/978-3-031-51458-6

This Springer imprint is published by the registered company Springer Nature Switzerland AG
The registered company address is: Gewerbestrasse 11, 6330 Cham, Switzerland

Paper in this product is recyclable.

S. Thikkurissy—To my loving Karin, you are amazing. Your impact on my heart and soul cannot be overstated. And to Bobban, whose face I see in every patient I care for.

S. Golkari—To my parents who brought me into medicine, William for seeing me through this journey and Dr. Kanchan Ganda who led by the example I wanted to follow.

Prologue: Conducting, Interpreting and Understanding the History and Physical: A Dentists Perspective

Sedation is a process-driven procedure. Independent of medication regimen used, how a sedation is accomplished should be a standardized process that ensures safety. The key to a successful sedation is continuous and continual assessment of the patient. This is accomplished through vital signs, visual assessment, and knowledge of typical pharmacodynamics of the regimen used.

This textbook will focus on the 'front end' of the sedation procedure, namely the pre-sedation assessment, the history and physical exam (H&P). Computer science uses the axiom 'Garbage in, Garbage out' (GIGO) to relate the importance of data input in the ultimate result. Similarly, a poorly done H&P leads to poor understanding of the patient, potentially placing the patient in a dangerous position. At times, there seems to be a focus on the litigious background with sedation and 'liability'. It is imperative to note that a physician-based H&P, up to 30 days prior to the sedation, offers questionable 'legal protection'. It is the responsibility of the sedating practitioner to assess the history and physical status on the day of sedation to not only assess changes, but also the veracity of a physician-based H&P. While this does diminish the value of the physician-based H&P, it rests on the adage 'Trust but verify'.

Therefore, this textbook will approach the H&P as something the sedating dentist should feel comfortable assessing. Additionally, the term 'directed H&P' will be used throughout the book to suggest an H&P that goes beyond general assessment to provide specific respiratory (or other system) recommendations. The American Academy of Pediatrics/American Academy of Pediatric Dentistry Joint sedation best practice document states: Before sedation, a health evaluation shall be performed by an appropriately licensed practitioner and reviewed by the sedation team at the time of treatment for possible interval changes [1]. This statement is open to interpretation due to the fact that this statement is intended for all sedation of children (under 18). The phrase 'appropriately licensed practitioner' may refer to the paediatric dentist. It is critical to note that the sedating team is expected to be able to review and assess the child on the day of sedation.

The standard for H&P 'expiration' is 30 days. The literature on this seems to be scant and seems to be more convention and self-referencing national guidelines. Having said that, 30 days seems to be a reasonable amount of time to avoid significant history and medical changes. It is important to note that many things can change within the span of those 30 days, and therefore it is the practitioner's job to reassess the patient prior to procedure even with the H&P present.

This textbook is organized by organ system and is intended to give dentists a practical algorithmic approach to assessing patient health and recognizing red flags as to require further consultation and directed questioning of physician colleagues.

Reference

1. American Academy of Pediatrics/American Academy of Pediatric Dentistry. Guidelines for monitoring and management of pediatric patients before, during, and after sedation for diagnostic and therapeutic procedures. Pediatrics. 2019;143(6):e20191000.

Chicago, IL
Cincinnati, OH

Sara Golkari
S. Thikkurissy

Contents

Conducting a History and Physical: "Succinct yet Exhaustive"

Sara Golkari and S. Thikkurissy

"The journey of a thousand miles begins with a single step." Lao Tzu

Once a patient has been selected for procedural sedation, the "single step" will be the history and physical workup. This textbook will not address selecting which patients to sedate, but rather, once those criteria have been set, this book will walk you through how to methodically approach assessing the history and physical of your patient. A graphic representation of elements of the H&P is noted in Fig. 1.1.

1. Standard Documentation: There are many different types of documentation for a history and physical (H&P). Particularly in a busy community pediatric dental practice, the H&P documentation may be subject to what forms community pediatric medical providers use. The Llack of standardization among forms can lead to differences in patient assessment. Parikh et al. [1] studying bariatric surgery noted that surgeons who used fully standardized forms had higher rates of documenting seven predetermined comorbidities compared to surgeons who did not use standardized (98% versus 74%, $P < 0.001$). The American Academy of Pediatric Dentistry (AAPD) does have a suggested standard sedation form that

S. Golkari
Philadelphia, PA, USA

S. Thikkurissy (✉)
Cincinnati Children's Hospital, Cincinnati, OH, USA
e-mail: Sarat.thikkurissy@cchmc.org

S. Thikkurissy, S. Golkari (eds.), *History and Physical for the Pediatric Dental Patient*, https://doi.org/10.1007/978-3-031-51458-6_1

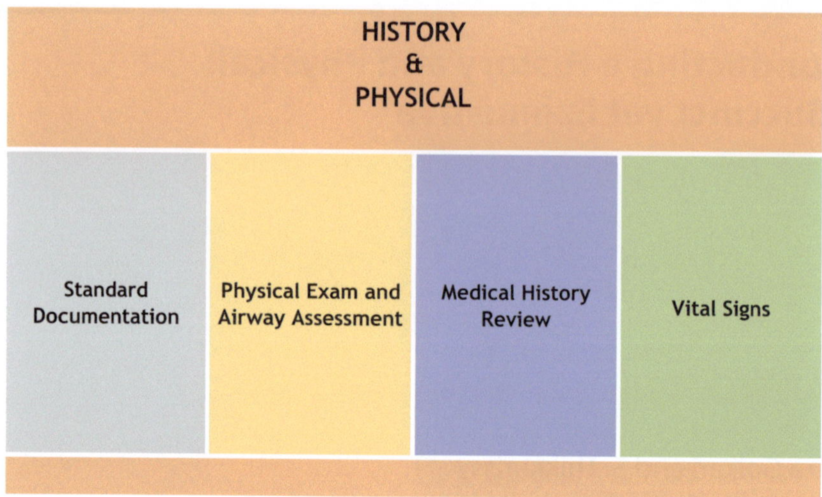

Fig. 1.1 Components of an H&P

includes an in-depth history and physical section, specifically targeting head and neck morbidities (including respiratory). This for can be obtained at aapd.org and searching for "'sedation."

Using a standardized form will allow for practitioners to be consistent in evaluating a patient. Convention is most situations is that the H&P is accomplished within 30 days of the procedural sedation. It should be noted that the further out from the sedation the H&P is accomplished, the less reliable and applicable it may be. That is to say, an H&P done 1 week out will be a more accurate representation of current health status than one done 28 days out. The Center for Medicaid Services (CMS) states: "The timeframe for completion of the H&P is no more than 30 days before or 24 hours after an admission. (Note: The term "admission" is used broadly to apply to either an admission as an inpatient or an admission to an outpatient service for which an H&P is required.) When the H&P is completed within 30 days before admission, an examination to determine any changes in the patient's current condition is to be completed and documented or entered into the medical record within 24 h of admission or prior to surgery or other procedures that you have deemed requires completion of an H&P' [2].

Some practitioners may require the patient's physician to complete the form prior to treatment. However, it should be noted that as the American Society of Anesthesiologists does, Practice Guidelines for Sedation and Analgesia by Non-Anesthesiologists states:

Clinicians administering sedation/analgesia should be familiar with sedation-oriented aspects of the patient's medical history and how these might alter the patient's response to sedation/analgesia. These include (1) abnormalities of the major organ systems; (2) previous adverse experience with sedation/analgesia as well as regional and general anesthesia;

(3) drug allergies, current medications, and potential drug interactions; (4) time and nature of last oral intake; and (5) history of tobacco, alcohol, or substance use or abuse. Patients presenting for sedation/analgesia should undergo a focused physical examination, including vital signs, auscultation of the heart and lungs, and evaluation of the airway [3].

Therefore, it is the responsibility of the sedating practitioner to wholly assess and document the patient's health on the day of sedation. A critical obstacle to properly assessing the patient is his/her behavior. This can be done by observing patient's behavior or play behavior in the waiting room [4]. A patient's behavior may be prohibitive or further complicate how accurately you may be able to evaluate the criteria listed on the H&P form including vital sign readings. Therefore, it is important to note patient's behavior at the time of intake.

2. Integration of Vital Sign Readings: The practitioner will be taking vital signs on the day of the sedation to assess physiologic health. This is particularly challenging with children, as behavioral responses can confound true vital sign readings, particularly in young children (three and under). The practitioner has to be able to integrate vital sign readings to get a baseline picture of where the child "'physiologically lives." This allows the sedating team to be able to understand how medications are affecting the child. It is a convention that otherwise young children who are obstreperous and unable to cooperate for vital sign collection may be documented as "UTO" (unable to obtain). This does however place the sedation dentist at a disadvantage as intraoperative vital signs may have limited context. If able to be obtained, baseline vital sign readings should include:

(a) Oxygen saturation—The resting oxygen saturation (SpO2) level should be assessed. This may be subject to patient core temperature, movement/crying, use of nail polish (particularly blue and black), and true physiologic low saturation. If the patient's baseline trends are relatively low (below 98%), it is incumbent upon provider to explain the low resting level prior to proceeding with the sedation. The concern is that a low resting level may suggest an acute or chronic airway issue that may become more prominent during sedation procedure.

Age (years)	Heart rate (beats/min) $\pm$ 2 SD
1–2 years	110 ± 40
2–4 years	105 ± 35
4–6 years	105 ± 35
6–12 years	95 ± 30
12–18 years	82 ± 25

(b) Heart rate—A baseline heart rate is recorded in beats per minute (BPM). The validity of this reading is subject to patient behavior including crying and anxiety. Practitioners should have awareness and access to a table of age-appropriate findings. Abnormal findings in this area would include patients with baseline bradycardia (American Heart Association definition <60 bpm), or a resting supraventricular tachycardia (>220 bpm). In a cooperative patient, this finding is of particular significance in that there typically is no behavior driving the elevated heart rate. Tachycardia can be found in increasingly stressful or exciting situations. Reading the baseline heart rate may also help distinguish between a sinus tachycardia: a very common situation-based elevation versus an organic arrhythmic dysfunction such as supraventricular tachycardia. A special word should be mentioned regarding bradycardia, or low heart rate. Bradycardia is an ominous reading and a potential precursor to fatal arrhythmia in the sedated patient. It is here that the decision-making of the practitioner is critical. Sedating a patient who presents with baseline bradycardia, particularly targeting moderate or deep sedation, may predispose the patient to arrhythmia.

(c) Blood pressure: Blood pressure readings may be closely related to heart rate findings and also related to nil per os (NPO)—fasting status. A patient who has been fasting for an extended period (beyond the recommended 8 h) may present as hypotensive. Again, an age-based chart will give some sense of context for appropriate age-based norms. A hypotensive patient may present with tachycardia, as the heart may compensate for hypotension/low blood pressure by elevating heart rate. Another way to measure hydration status/risk for hypotension is through use of the capillary refill. To assess the patient's capillary refill time, press on the finger for 5 s using moderate pressure at room temperature (20–25 °C) and count how long it takes for the finger to regain its original color. A capillary refill time of 2–3 s is considered normal.

(d) Auscultation—Chapters 5 and 6 will address the specifics of cardiac and pulmonary auscultation. This is an essential part of the pre-sedation workup that may be challenging in a child who is unable to cooperate due to age and/or developmental status.

3. Medical History Review: The review of the patient's medical history is a familiar area for dental practitioners as this is typically done with every appointment. Due to the nature of the sedation procedure, the H&P should be "succinct yet exhaustive." Specific details about medical problems, medications, allergies, and surgical history should be addressed. Additionally, there should be material about recent history of emergency room/urgent care visits. Specifically of interest would be whether these visits were for respiratory-based illnesses. Related to this, recent illness that could impact airway (e.g., upper respiratory infection, croup) may affect airway reactivity with certain sedation medications, and sedation should be deferred approximately 4–6 weeks following resolution of symptoms (assuming no hospitalization is required). It is important to always review medical history even in the presence of already provided history from general physician as sometimes omissions may be present from the original records given.

For younger children (three and under), birth history can be particularly significant. Gestation term, prematurity, and comorbidities such as neonatal intubations, need for supplemental oxygen therapy, and surfactant delivery are critical in creating a picture of a patient's neonatal health. For instance, bronchopulmonary dysplasia is a lung disease, which can result from long-term hyperoxygenation and is strongly associated with prematurity and early airway morbidity [5]. These perinatal morbidities can significantly affect whether a patient is an acceptable or poor sedation candidate.

The medication review should include specific medication names, dosages, and time of day medications taken as some medications (such as seasonal allergy medications) may have an additive depressive effect when combined with sedatives. Additionally, if patient needs to take medication with food, this should be considered consistent with ASA NPO guidelines.

4. Physical Exam and Airway Assessment: The core of this book will be a systems-based assessment of the patient, including strategies for physical exam. It must be underscored that despite pre-sedation H&P, a day of workup/review must be completed, including a physical exam (to include airway assessment). An example of the importance of the day-of- sedation exam relates specifically to tonsil size. While a child may present with tonsillar obstruction of the airway of less than 25% 2 weeks in advance of the sedation, the day of presentation is subject to a recent history of illness, so there may be greater obstruction of the airway. Similarly, depending on the time of the year sedations are conducted, children may be at higher risk of developing respiratory viral infections between presedation workup and day of procedure. The burden of responsibility lies on the practitioner conducting the sedation to confirm that patient is still a viable candidate for sedation

This text will review how to include elements from key organ systems into the presedation history and physical and when it is best to defer sedation or refer for further evaluation. The following chapters will dive into specific organ systems that will be addressed in your H&P in a systematic approach.

References

1. Parikh JA, Yermilov I, Jain S, et al. How much do standardized forms improve the documentation of quality of care? J Surg Res. 2007;143(1):158–63.
2. Implications of CMS Changes to H&P Requirements. https://www.hcpro.com/ACC-65354-1000/Implications-of-CMS-Changes-to-HP-Requirements.html. Accessed 2 Apr 2021.
3. American Society Anesthesiologists. Practice guidelines for sedation and analgesia by non-anesthesiologists. Anesthesiology. 2017.
4. McTigue DJ, Pinkham J. Association between children's dental behavior and play behavior. ASDC J Dent Child. 1978;45(3):218–22.
5. O'Brodovich HM, Steinhorn R, Ward RM, Hallman M, Schwartz EJ, Vanya M, Janssen EM, Mangili A, Han L, Sarda SP. Development of a severity scale to assess chronic lung disease after extremely preterm birth. Pediatr Pulmonol. 2021;56(6):1583–92.

Assessment of the Vital Signs

2

S. Thikkurissy

Vital signs are tools used by the practitioner to reflect the health status of the patient. They give relative "guard rails" for the practitioner to be aware of to avoid putting extreme physiologic strain on the patient. In pediatrics, this understanding is even more critical because vital sign fluctuation is age related. As children grow, there are increases in quantity and quality of alveoli for gas exchange, anatomic changes in muscle tone, diaphragmatic anatomy, and vascular resistance among other variables. With regard to procedural sedation, it should be remembered that, as noted by Mazzeo, "The level at which an increase in carbon dioxide tension is tolerated without complication depends on many variables, such as, age concomitant diseases, the speed at which high values are reached and the duration of supercarbia" [1]. Mazzeo goes on to note that children due to overall lower oxygen reserves and reduced functional (pulmonary) capacities are at greater risk of hypercarbia. This rate of carbon dioxide increase is greater in children due to their metabolic rate relation to both weight and oxygen reserve. In layman's terms these findings reflect a key underlining principle in pediatric procedural sedation, namely, children demonstrate less physiologic compensation for respiratory compromise. This means that the practitioner must be able to integrate vital sign readings real time with how the patient is responding in terms of effective ventilation and resultant oxygenation. A caveat before proceeding, vital signs are subject to behavior, and in some instances the obstreperous nature of the child will lead to abnormal vital sign readings; the practitioner needs to be able to integrate the clinical situation as well as the vital readings and make an informed decision, shared with caregivers, whether it is safe to proceed with the sedation.

In this chapter we will focus not on the actual vital sign monitors, but when in the course of the history and physical, further consultation may be warranted and procedural sedation deferred.

S. Thikkurissy (✉)
Cincinnati Children's Hospital, Cincinnati, OH, USA
e-mail: Sarat.thikkurissy@cchmc.org

© The Author(s), under exclusive license to Springer Nature Switzerland AG 2023
S. Thikkurissy, S. Golkari (eds.), *History and Physical for the Pediatric Dental Patient*, https://doi.org/10.1007/978-3-031-51458-6_2

2.1 Development of the Lung

While development of the lung can be divided into the embryonic, fetal, and postnatal periods, the timing of this development is of utmost interest in procedural sedation. It is during the postnatal period that alveolarization begins and continues throughout childhood growth. Indeed, Schittny points out that microvascular maturation and growth of alveolar capillaries (where gas exchange occurs) is observed between 36 weeks of growth and 21 years [2].

Therefore, it is critical to understand that there is a developmental increase in both the quality and quantity of surface areas for gas exchange in the lungs. The classic postnatal alveolarization process is seen when new septa divide off from existing septa and form airspaces/alveoli. It is critical for practitioners to realize that prematurity may significantly impact pulmonary development, as well as reducing surface area for gas exchange. Placing a previously premature infant under moderate to deep procedural sedation may result in respiratory depression from which the child will be unable to recover. Therefore, it is imperative, particularly with young children (2–3 years of age) that a birth history is obtained. Issues such as extreme prematurity/very low birth weight, postnatal intubation, and need for supplemental oxygen therapy in infancy or early childhood all need to be accounted for when deciding if procedural sedation is appropriate and which regimens one might use when proceeding.

2.2 Sleep Disordered Breathing

Another important area of evaluation of the patient should be sleep behavior as it may provide clues to a more serious ventilation issue in the child. A key concept to understand when working a patient up for procedural sedation is that of sleep-disordered breathing (SDB). Statistics put SDB as a feature in up to 3% of children [3]. SDB may be secondary to an obstruction such as hypertrophic tonsils, or larger than normal macroglossia. Secondary to this obstruction, oxygen levels may fall, and carbon dioxide levels rise. This triggers a gasp or waking to take a breath. This is known as obstructive sleep apnea as compared to central sleep apnea in which pathophysiology is related to a central nervous system defect that may include the brainstem and the generation of respiration. While there is a relationship between SDB and obesity, there is also a relationship observed in children with significant prematurity/failure to thrive. Signs of SDB may include snoring, waking up choking or even vomiting, and in older children particularly daytime somnolence noted typically in school [3]. There have also been associations noted between SDB/OSA and enuresis (bedwetting) in children older than 1 year. The practitioner who is working a child up for procedural sedation should be asking about sleep habits including regular bedtime and disruptions during sleep. It is also important to ask about behavioral "combativeness" in going to sleep. The reason for this is that as some sedative regimens are used to promote sleep, a child that "fights" going to sleep may be unrestful and procedural sedation may not be the best method of treatment.

The vital sign that is most often associated with ventilation is capnography and uses the end-tidal CO_2 measurement to quantify respiratory health. As mentioned above, it is critical to remember that in most adverse situations, a problem with ventilation will likely occur before the problem with oxygenation.

2.3 Mechanism of Gas Exchange

As mentioned earlier, microvascular maturation occurs from 36 weeks in utero to 21 years postnatal. The development of the capillaries that allow gas exchange are seen to proceed parallel to the development of the alveoli. During approximately in utero week 24 to birth, there is a process forming sacculi which will result in future surface areas for gas exchange. The pulmonary septa during development possess a double-layered capillary network which is ultimately responsible for gas exchange, but not before it will fuse into a single-layered capillary network contained within the septum [3]. Having an understanding and appreciation of pulmonary development allows the practitioner to see how early childhood illness can impact gas exchange as well as the child's ability to compensate during obstruction episodes intraoperatively. The vital sign most associated with oxygenation is the pulse oximeter/oxygen saturation reading. It is critical to remember that oximetry readings are subject to delay and may not give an immediate detection of an apneic episode as capnography will.

2.4 Abnormal Vital Sign Readings

During the course of the workup, the practitioner may come across an abnormal vital sign reading. It is at this time that the most valuable monitor (the practitioners' intellect and understanding) come into play. The practitioner will need to determine if the aberrance is due to child's behavior or true organic abnormality. A commonly held convention is that the more disruptive the child, the less true the child's vital signs. Many practitioners who conclude it is safe to proceed will note "UTO" or "unable to obtain due to behavior" on their sedation record. It is ultimately the practitioner's risk assessment that allow them to proceed without all the information. Likewise, the less disruptive and calmer the child, the more the vital sign reading may indeed be accurate and abnormal. This is where the practitioner will need to refer to their primary care colleague for a more in-depth assessment.

Vital sign assessments are critical in providing surrogate measures for the child's overall health and safety to proceed with the procedural sedation and his/her stability intraoperatively. Having the ability to properly obtain, assess, and monitor a patient's vital signs preoperatively, intraoperatively, and postoperatively will allow practitioners to act accordingly in order to minimize patient risk.

References

1. Mazzeo A, Spada A, Pratico C, et al. Hypercapnia: what is the limit in paediatric patients? A case of near-fatal asthma successfully treated by multipharmacological approach. Pediatr Anesth. 2004;14:596–603.
2. Schittny JC. Development of the lung. Cell Tissue Res. 2017;367(3):427–44.
3. Pediatric Sleep-disordered Breathing. https://www.childrens.com/specialties-services/conditions/sleep-disorder-breathing. Accessed 11 Nov 2021.

Assessment of the Head and Neck

3

S. Thikkurissy

A methodical approach to any examination is always encouraged, and the head and neck region is no different. A straightforward way of assessment can be to split the physical exam into extraoral (EOE) and intraoral (IOE) examinations.

3.1 Extraoral Examination

The extraoral examination begins from the moment the practitioner sees the patient. Assessment of temperament, gait, or any deviations from "normal" can be noted in the waiting room and during the initial greeting. The practitioner will learn how to note asymmetries, condition of the hair, or gross dermatologic conditions such as eczema in this high-level assessment. Once the patient is seated and a more focused examination is occurring, the EOE can target areas of the head neck such as the scalp, ears, and nose and should note any abrasions, contusions, or swellings. Any perceived deviations from normal can be discussed with the guardian during the history portion of the H&P as well and should be properly documented. Over time, the EOE will become part of the initial survey on any patient encountered. Typically, an abnormality noted on the EOE will be referred to the primary care physician and based on the severity of aberrance may result in a cancelled procedural sedation.

3.2 Differential Considerations for Deviations: Child Abuse

A physical exam on a child cannot be discussed responsibly without bringing up the differential diagnosis of child abuse. The peak age of child abuse and neglect is in the preverbal population and peaking at 2–3 years. Another group that is at high risk

S. Thikkurissy (✉)
Cincinnati Children's Hospital, Cincinnati, OH, USA
e-mail: Sarat.thikkurissy@cchmc.org

© The Author(s), under exclusive license to Springer Nature Switzerland AG 2023
S. Thikkurissy, S. Golkari (eds.), *History and Physical for the Pediatric Dental Patient*, https://doi.org/10.1007/978-3-031-51458-6_3

are those with special health needs, particularly when impacting mobility and verbal communication. Anytime a dentist is conducting a physical exam, particularly on a child, they need to be aware and cognizant of intentional injuries. The most common areas this might appear include behind the ear and inside the mouth (frenal attachments, buccal mucosa). A few pathognomonic injuries to consider include:

(a) Raccoon's sign (bilateral black eyes with history of single blow)
(b) Battle's sign (ecchymosis on the mastoid process behind ear)
(c) Injury in the so-called danger triangle of the neck, the area bordered by the sternocleidomastoid muscle, which is normally protected during injury.

All healthcare providers are typically mandated providers (see specific state/country Department of Health or equivalent for details), and so if any suspicious injuries are noted, or there is inconsistency between the injury and the story from guardian as to how the injury occurred, reporting is required.

3.3 Examination of the Neck

The neck is not only critical for the structures it houses but additionally its proximity to the airway. Diseases of the neck may result in tracheal deviation and/or airway compromise. Examination of the neck is best undertaken with the child reclined in the dental chair with the chin tilted up. This allows clear view without the child's head position obstructing view. Aside from gross asymmetry, the neck should be examined for potential lymphadenopathy along the cervical and submandibular regions. Lymphadenopathy may be associated with transient illness but may also be secondary to facial cellulitis in which there may be tracking down the side of the neck resulting in either lymphadenopathy or lymphadenitis. It is important to observe the neck range of motion, particularly in instances where there is lymph-related swelling, or asymmetry. A limited range of motion may result in a hindered ability to rescue the airway if needed. Additionally, if the range of motion limitation includes rigidity/tenderness at the posterior skull (nuchal rigidity), this warrants an urgent referral to the child's primary care provider for immediate assessment, as meningitis is within the differential considerations.

In addition to lateral assessment of the neck and range of motion, the dentist should also make note of the thyromental distance. The thyromental distance is the distance from the chin to the top of the notch of the thyroid cartilage. This will give some idea of the retrognathic positioning of the mandible and how effective an emergency rescue maneuver such as the jaw thrust will be. Patients with a short thyromental distance may have a "setback" (retrognathic) mandible that can be challenging to position forward with a jaw thrust. Coupling this with a young child's relative macroglossia and a typical flatter mandibular plane angle is suggestive that the airway may obstruct easier than in a child without those variables.

3.4   Obesity

Obesity in pediatric population is defined by the Centers for Disease Control and Prevention (CDC) as at or above the 95th percentile compared to other children/teens. Since a child's body composition varies not only between ages, but also between genders, a comparative percentile is used versus the whole number system used for adults. It is critical to note that while BMI is highly correlative with other measures of body fat such as skinfold thickness measurements, BMI does *not* measure body fat directly. Therefore, the distribution of body fat also needs to be considered [1]. Android body fat is primarily located surrounding the chest and stomach areas. This is particularly of concern during procedural sedation as it can contribute to restriction of respiratory effort (especially if protective stabilization such as a papoose board, Pedi-Wrap, Joey Board, etc. are used). Gynoid obesity is most noted around the hips and thighs and is typically less seen in children. Ovoid obesity is the most even distribution of adipose tissue and should be evaluated with the same eye as android obesity and the upper airway. Distribution should also be noted regarding the neck and pressure placed from redundant adipose.

3.5   Intraoral Examination

The IOE is something that most dentists will be familiar with and thus will be dealt with in an abbreviated manner. There will likely be (due to the need for procedural sedation) dental caries. There may also be newly erupted and/or exfoliating teeth depending on the child's dental age. These should be assessed in treatment planning the sedation, but also critically the day of the sedation, as they are potential sources for airway obstruction during a sedation. It is critical to remember that as the level of sedation gets deeper, there is a decreased functioning in the protective reflexes, and so a normally minor concern such as an exfoliating tooth may become dislodged and obstruct the airway.

3.6   Tonsils

Tonsillar tissue serves as part of the immune response and function within the lymphatic system. There are four groupings of tonsils: palatine, lingual, adenoid, and nasopharyngeal. The last two will serve as particularly critical in the presedation assessment. The adenoid and nasopharyngeal tonsils may be hypertrophic due to both acute and chronic illness such as sinusitis and otitis media. The most common scale used to identify tonsil size and/or impingement on the airway is the Brodsky scale. In the Brodsky scale, the amount of available airway that is obstructed by tonsillar tissue is evaluated. The scale ranges from 0 (tonsils are absent or have been removed) to 4 (in which the tonsils occupy more than 75% of the available airway). These extreme cases are colloquially called "kissing tonsils" because the right and left tonsils meet at the midline. It is critical to understand that whatever the presedation assessment is in terms of tonsillar obstruction will worsen once the child is sedated. Relaxation of the tensor veli palatini and the pharyngeal wall typically results in midline migration of tonsils in a sedated airway. For instance, a patient is a Brodsky 3 preoperative (50–75% obstruction) may become a Brodsky 4 (>75% obstruction) upon sedation.

It should be noted that in younger children, the relative macroglossia may obstruct a clear view of the tonsils. In this case, it may be necessary for the practitioner to depress the tongue with a mirror or tongue blade and cause a momentary "gag." The importance of assessing tonsils the day of sedation cannot be overstated. Once a patient is sedated, and tissues in the oropharynx potentially relax, redundant tissues in the posterior oropharynx and tonsillar tissue will deviate to the midline causing increased risk for obstruction. For instance, a child who is assessed to have 50–75% tonsillar obstruction (Brodsky 3) presedation may become a 75% (Brodsky 4) or greater postsedation depending on the regimen used and the individual response to the medications. In many cases, tonsil size itself is not a "disqualifying" variable for procedural sedation (other than near 100% obstruction anecdotally known as "kissing tonsils") but may alter the choice of sedative regimen and doses to be used.

3.7 The Tongue

It is important to note that children have a tongue size: oropharynx size ratio when compared to adults. As noted earlier, this "relative" macroglossia in combination with a flatter mandibular plane leads to the tongue being the most common site of upper airway obstruction in the pediatric patient. When assessing the tongue, the relative "size" of the tongue to the oral cavity should be noted. While there is no finite scale for measuring tongue size in the pediatric patient, its obstruction of airway visualization is an adequate surrogate measure to consider.

The head and neck examination will be further discussed in subsequent chapters. It is a foundational exam due to the intersection of the airway and the site of work for dental treatment under procedural sedation.

Reference

1. Barlow SE, the Expert Committee. Expert committee recommendations regarding the prevention, assessment, and treatment of child and adolescent overweight and obesity: summary report. Pediatrics. 2007;120:S164–92.

The Eye Examination During a Dental Procedure

Eniolami O. Dosunmu

4.1 The Examination

4.1.1 Vision

A vision examination is dependent on the age of the child and must be developmentally appropriate. Obtaining a vision prior to procedural sedation/anesthesia is not indicated, unless there is a concern that a baseline vision prior to procedural intervention is of importance and will have bearing on the postoperative outcome. In such settings, a formal vision should be obtained by an ophthalmologist. In circumstances where this is not possible, an assessment of vision should be obtained prior to the procedure by the dentist. An age-appropriate eye chart should be used. For children over the age 6 years, Sloan letters/Snellen eye chart is recommended. For children ages 3–5, use of LEA symbols® or HOTV letters is recommended. In preverbal or nonverbal children, preferential looking cards can be used for a vision assessment. Observation for whether there is a preference for one eye over the other is also another avenue, to assess vision. It may not always be accurate but is a quick evaluation tool. Knowing whether there was previous amblyopia, or vision loss, or if there is a need for refractive correction will be helpful during this assessment.

4.1.2 Pupils

The pupil examination is very important, as this will provide information about the integrity of the eye and also provides neurologic information. It is important to assess for whether the pupils are equal in size, reactive to light—both the direct and consensual response—and round in shape.

E. O. Dosunmu (✉)
Cincinnati Children's Hospital, Cincinnati, OH, USA
e-mail: Eniolami.dosunmu@cchmc.org

Performing a pupil examination: Using a light source, the size of each pupil is determined, ensuring that both are equal in size. Next, the light is shone into one eye, and the reaction of the pupil is observed (a normal reaction is for pupil constriction), the light is then shone in the contralateral eye, looking for the same response (constriction of the pupil in that eye). Next, the light is shone into each eye—going back and forth—as the examiner swings the light source between both eyes; a normal finding is constriction of the pupils. In the presence of a relative afferent pupil defect, when the light is shone from the unaffected eye to the affected eye, the pupils of both eyes will be noted to dilate.

A well-documented history will be helpful to determine if there is a previous anisocoria (unequal pupil sizes) or altered anatomy to the iris that would result in changes in the pupil shape, or previous optic nerve or neurologic injury that would result in a relative afferent pupillary defect.

4.1.3 Lids, Lashes, and Orbit

An external evaluation of the eyelids, the eyelashes, and the periorbital and orbital areas for any preexisting anatomical changes is important prior to any procedural sedation/anesthesia and prior to any dental procedure. External examination may also reveal infectious processes that would negate proceeding with procedural sedation and a dental procedure, for example, herpes simplex infection with active vesicles on the face, or in the periorbital area. It could also reveal changes suggestive of an active neurologic process, for example, a new-onset ptosis (droopy eyelid), or a facial droop that may necessitate deferment.

4.1.4 Motility

Motility of the extraocular muscles should demonstrate normal excursions of the extraocular muscles in the absence of previous ophthalmic disease such as trauma, known restrictive strabismus such as thyroid eye disease, known paralytic strabismus, or other orbital process. Assessment of extraocular motility may be important, post-procedure, in localizing, if there is a concern for an inadvertent ophthalmic complication/neurologic complication.

4.2 Sclera and Conjunctiva

The sclera and conjunctiva are typically white in color. Changes in the color may be suggestive of systemic illness, e.g., in jaundice there is a yellow discoloration to the sclera, and local trauma, e.g., a subconjunctival hemorrhage, or infection. The presence of an active conjunctivitis may warrant delay of the dental procedure.

4.2.1 Cornea

Examination of the cornea should demonstrate a clear "window" into the anterior chamber of the eye with no opacity/cloudiness/haze of the cornea. This is also a good time to evaluate for the use of contact lenses, which may need to be removed prior to procedural sedation/anesthesia. It is important to ensure proper closure of the eyes for the entirety of the procedure to ensure no corneal abrasions. It is recommended that an ophthalmic lubricating ointment/tears be placed, followed by manual eyelid closure to ensure no lagophthalmos (incomplete eyelid closure), and this is secured with the use of medical-grade tape.

4.2.2 Anterior Chamber

The anterior chamber is the space between the cornea and the iris plane. The use of a penlight/light source will be useful in determining the depth of the anterior chamber. When light is shone from the temporal aspect of the eye toward the nasal aspect, if the light can be seen nasally, the anterior is determined to the deep [1].

4.2.3 Red Reflex

Using a direct ophthalmoscope, one can identify the red reflex in the eyes. In the absence of strabismus, media opacity, and retinal or optic nerve disease, the red reflex should be symmetric in both eyes. The presence of a white or absent reflex in a child, with no known previous history, should warrant immediate ophthalmologic evaluation.

4.2.4 Eye Reflexes

There are several eye reflexes of importance that once should be knowledgeable of during procedural sedation/anesthesia for dental procedures/surgeries. These are discussed below.

Pupillary light reflex: This was discussed above. This reflex may be disrupted in the setting of anesthesia [2].

Oculocardiac reflex: This reflex results in a decrease in the resting heart rate when there is stimulation of the eye, orbit, or the extraocular muscles—usually through stretching of the extraocular muscles [2, 3]. This is more prominent in the pediatric population, where a dramatic drop in the heart rate can be seen.

Corneal reflex: Tactile stimulation of the cornea results in blinking of both eyes [3].

Lacrimatory reflex/reflex lacrimation: This is tearing/lacrimation in response to various stimuli—stimuli to the cornea, conjunctiva, and nasal mucosa, bright lights, emotional upset, vomiting, coughing, and emesis [2, 3].

Gusto-lacrimal reflex/crocodile tear syndrome: Unilateral lacrimation that occurs during eating or drinking [3, 4]. This is typically seen after facial trauma or Bell's palsy.

Bell's phenomenon: Upward deviation of the eyes during eyelid closure against resistance [2]. This reflex is present in 90% of the population [2, 3]. This can be absent in some local eye disease processes, such as an entrapped muscle from orbital trauma.

Oculo-respiratory reflex: This results in a decrease in the respiratory rate, shallow breathing, or respiratory arrest when pressure is placed on the eye or orbit or when the extraocular muscles are stretched. When under general anesthesia with mechanical ventilation, this is often not appreciated; however, manipulation of the eye/orbital structures under sedation should warrant close evaluation of the respiratory status [3, 5].

Oculo-emetic reflex: This results in increased nausea and emesis following extensive manipulation of the extraocular muscles [3]. This should be considered when dental and ophthalmic cases are combined, especially if the dental wounds are to be kept relatively dry.

4.3 Ophthalmic and Systemic Considerations Prior to Dental Procedures

There are several ophthalmic reasons to defer a dental procedure. One of those is an active infection periorbital and/or orbital process. An active herpes/varicella eruption that involves the orbital region or the facial region that has not been adequately treated is at risk for progression/systemic spread. An active preseptal inflammatory/infectious process and/or orbital cellulitis whose etiology is not dental is also at risk for progression/systemic spread. In an immune compromised patient, this could lead to dissemination in the setting of a dental procedure given the proximity to the orbits/facial structures and oral structures to one another. An active infectious, untreated, conjunctivitis is also another clinical indication to defer a dental procedure. An active keratitis is also a reason to defer a dental procedure, as these patients often need frequent topical application of topical antimicrobial medication that would contraindicate eye closure for the anesthesia. In addition, it is important to identify the source of the active infection, to ensure that it would also not result to a postoperative complication of the dental procedure/surgery. In the setting of an endophthalmitis, a dental procedure needs to be deferred, especially if the etiology of the endophthalmitis has not been elucidated. If it is an endogenous source (nondental source), this may also pose a risk for the dental procedure. In addition, in the setting of a compromised eye, without proper premedication with antimicrobials, as dental procedures are known to result in a transient septicemia, this could further compromise an already diseased eye.

Systemic diseases with ophthalmic manifestations should be accounted for when a dental procedure/surgery is to be performed, given the possible ophthalmic complications, and given the fact that known ophthalmic responses could mirror dental healing as both have mucous membranes. Diseases such as epidermolysis bullosa could result in corneal abrasions or corneal scarring if proper preventative measures are not taken during the procedural sedation/anesthesia. Other diseases such as systemic and ocular graft versus host disease, Sjogren's disease where the risk of ocular surface dryness is increased, and thyroid eye disease with proptosis with increased risk of dryness and decreased Bell's phenomenon could also result in ophthalmic complications. Previous refractive surgery results in increased keratoconjunctivitis sicca [6], and knowledge of this could help during the sedation/anesthesia when the ocular surface is being protected. This is also important if there is a chemical or body fluid exposure to the ocular surface, or if there is trauma to the ocular surface during instrumentation of the teeth, or from accidental ocular surface exposure, as treatment may need to be altered to account for the prior refractive surgery.

4.4 Dental Local Anesthesia and Potential Ophthalmic Complications

There are many studies that discuss ophthalmic complications of unintended spread of local anesthesia during dental procedures [7–13]. The exact mechanism of the spread has been debated in the medical literature—intra-arterial, intravenous, localized spread, incorrect anatomic location of injection, etc. A careful ophthalmic examination prior to the start of the sedation/anesthesia will be very helpful to determine what the acute changes are and how to best treat them. With the use of general anesthesia in the pediatric population, the use of local anesthesia/blocks may be decreased, and these rare complications may not arise. We will briefly discuss the potential findings/complications here: transient amaurosis (blindness), diplopia (double vision) with temporary paresis of one or more of the extraocular muscles, ptosis (drooping of the upper eyelid), mydriasis (dilation of the pupil), miosis (constriction of the pupil), nystagmus (involuntary movements of the eyes), and retrobulbar pain have been reported [7–11]. With the spread of the local anesthesia to the orbital space/into the ophthalmic circulation, the resulting findings are secondary to the anesthetic effect and/or to the vasoconstrictor effect, as most anesthetics are used in combination with a vasoconstrictor. These are rare complications, and even more rare are the reports of permanent vision loss in the setting of local anesthetic use, where irreversible damage occurs to the ophthalmic circulation that supplies the optic nerve and/or retina [12, 13].

4.5 General Anesthetic Agents and Intraocular Pressure Changes

Studies have demonstrated that the newer inhalation agents (sevoflurane, desflurane, and isoflurane) used for induction anesthesia decrease the measured intraocular pressure (IOP) [14–17]. Ketamine has been reported to either have no effect on the IOP or to increase the IOP [14, 16, 17]. Succinylcholine has been consistently shown to increase the IOP1 [4], and propofol has been shown to decrease the IOP [14]. The use of succinylcholine is generally avoided in an eye with an open globe/penetrating/perforating injury as the increase in IOP may result in expulsion of the intraocular contents.

Nitrous oxide is frequently used in combination with one of the abovementioned anesthetic agents for anesthesia in dental procedures/surgeries. One study, in healthy adults, found the use of nitrous oxide only, has no significant effect on IOP [18]. The use of nitrous oxide is contraindicated if there is an ophthalmic surgical history where recent intraocular gas was used. In such settings, the nitrous oxide can rapidly expand in the intraocular gas, thus raising the intraocular pressure and resulting in the occlusion of the central retinal artery. Unfortunately, this results in permanent vision loss [19, 20]. It is important to have a complete ophthalmic surgical history, as this knowledge will prevent such an outcome. Patients with intraocular gas bubbles are fitted with a bracelet that is to remain on until removed by the vitreoretinal surgeon, once the bubble is completely resorbed [19].

Another thing of note with recent vitreoretinal surgery is positioning of the patient. Patients are typically placed in certain positions, so that the intraocular gas can help tamponade a retinal tear/detachment during the healing phase. These positioning needs should be taken into consideration prior to any sedation/anesthesia as the positioning needed for the dental procedure/surgery may be contraindicated to that needed during the vitreoretinal surgery postoperative period. Most young pediatric patients cannot adhere to the positioning rules for the duration of the time that is needed following vitreoretinal surgery; thus, silicone oil is used as a tamponade instead [21]. It should be noted that when there is silicone oil in the eye, prolonged supine position will lead to silicone oil bubbles in the anterior chamber; however, with upright position or with a prone position, this easily resolves.

It is also important to ensure avoid hypotension during anesthesia, as prolonged hypotension could lead to decreased perfusion of the optic nerve and retina and result in irreversible vision loss [22, 23].

4.6 Potential Ophthalmic Complications from Dental Procedures

Corneal abrasions: These can result from chemical exposure, mechanical exposure (either from instrumentation or from debris), body fluid exposure, from ultraviolet light exposure (when lasers are used), or other traumas directly to the eye. Abrasions can also occur if the eyes were not carefully closed for the duration of the anesthesia, and the epithelial tissue degrades resulting in an abrasion. If the abrasion is inoculated with a microbe, a keratitis may result. An abrasion should be treated to ensure complete resolution with no long-term sequelae on vision. A keratitis in the setting of previous refractive surgery, especially laser-assisted in situ keratomileusis (LASIK), where a flap was created, can be difficult to treat, if the microbe inoculates tissue beneath the flap.

Corneal and conjunctival foreign bodies: These can result from debris from the dental procedures. The eyes should be flushed with eye wash or saline and the patient referred to ophthalmology for further evaluation.

Subconjunctival hemorrhage: A subconjunctival hemorrhage results when there is a broken blood vessel beneath the conjunctival layer of the eye. These result from direct trauma or from increased Valsalva maneuvers that result in rupture of the vessels [24].

Retinopathy: Constant exposure to ultraviolet lights (during the use of lasers) without the use of proper protective glasses may result in a retinopathy.

Periorbital and subcutaneous emphysema: This is a rare complication and occurs often during tooth extraction when high-powered drills are used, whereby compressed air is forced into the subcutaneous tissues [25–27]. A careful examination of the eye or orbit and surrounding facial structures should be used as a guide for treatment.

Endophthalmitis: This is a serious, but thankfully rare complication. This could result from direct inoculation [28] or endogenous spread [29] in a patient. Immediate ophthalmology care should be sought in the setting of an endophthalmitis.

Trauma: Any noted trauma warrants immediate ophthalmology evaluation. One of the more serious complications is an open globe injury that needs immediate surgical intervention.

References

1. American Academy of Ophthalmology. Penlight examination of chamber angle. https://www.aao.org/image/penlight-examination-of-chamber-angle.
2. Hunyor AP. Reflexes and the eye. Aust N Z J Ophthalmol. 1994;22:155–9. https://doi.org/10.1111/j.1442-9071.1994.tb01710.x.
3. EyeWiki, American Academy of Ophthalmology. Reflexes and the eye. https://eyewiki.aao.org/Reflexes_and_the_Eye#cite_note-14.
4. Montoya FJ, Riddell CE, Caesar R, Hague S. Treatment of gustatory hyperlacrimation (crocodile tears) with injection of botulinum toxin into the lacrimal gland. Eye (Lond). 2002;16(6):705–9. https://doi.org/10.1038/sj.eye.6700230.
5. Blanc VF, Jacob JL, Milot J, et al. The oculorespiratory reflex revisited. Can J Anaesth. 1988;35:468. https://doi.org/10.1007/BF03026892.
6. Ang RT, Dartt DA, Tsubota K. Dry eye after refractive surgery. Curr Opin Ophthalmol. 2001;12(4):318–22. https://doi.org/10.1097/00055735-200108000-00013.
7. Steenen SA, Dubois L, Saeed P, de Lange J. Ophthalmologic complications after intraoral local anesthesia: case report and review of literature. Oral Surg Oral Med Oral Pathol Oral Radiol. 2012;113:e1–5.
8. Pragasm M, Managutti A. Diplopia with local anesthesia. Natl J Maxillofac Surg. 2011;2(1):82–5. https://doi.org/10.4103/0975-5950.85861.
9. Ko IC, Park KS, Shin JM, Baik JS. Visual loss after intraoral local anesthesia for the removal of circumzygomatic and circum-mandibular wires: a case report. J Oral Maxillofac Surg. 2015;73(10):1918.e1–1918.e19186. https://doi.org/10.1016/j.joms.2015.06.178.
10. Horowitz J, Almog Y, Wolf A, Buckman G, Geyer O. Ophthalmic complications of dental anesthesia: three new cases. J Neuroophthalmol. 2005;25(2):95–100.

11. Wilkie GJ. Temporary uniocular blindness and ophthalmoplegia associated with a mandibular block injection. A case report. Aust Dent J. 2000;45(2):131–3. https://doi.org/10.1111/j.1834-7819.2000.tb00253.

12. Oğurel T, Onaran Z, Oğurel R, Örnek N, Büyüktortop Gökçınar N, Örnek K. Branch retinal artery occlusion following dental extraction. Case Rep Ophthalmol Med. 2014;2014:202834. https://doi.org/10.1155/2014/202834.

13. Khattab MH, Wiegand A, Storch M, Hoerauf H, Feltgen N. Unilateral vision loss after a dental visit. Case Rep Ophthalmol. 2018;9(1):204–9. https://doi.org/10.1159/000487586.

14. Mikhail M, Sabri K, Levin AV. Effect of anesthesia on intraocular pressure measurement in children. Surv Ophthalmol. 2017;62(5):648–58. https://doi.org/10.1016/j.survophthal.2017.04.003.

15. Runciman JC, Bowen-Wright RM, Welsh NH, Downing JW. Intra-ocular pressure changes during halothane and enflurance anaesthesia. Br J Anaesth. 1978;50(4):371–4. https://doi.org/10.1093/bja/50.4.371.

16. Jones L, Sung V, Lascaratos G, Nagi H, Holder R. Intraocular pressures after ketamine and sevoflurane in children with glaucoma undergoing examination under anaesthesia. Br J Ophthalmol. 2010;94(1):33–5. https://doi.org/10.1136/bjo.2008.148122.

17. Blumberg D, Congdon N, Jampel H, et al. The effects of sevoflurane and ketamine on intraocular pressure in children during examination under anesthesia. Am J Ophthalmol. 2007;143(3):494–9. https://doi.org/10.1016/j.ajo.2006.11.061.

18. Lalwani K, Fox EB, Fu R, Edmunds B, Kelly LD. The effect of nitrous oxide on intra-ocular pressure in healthy adults. Anaesthesia. 2012;67(3):256–60. https://doi.org/10.1111/j.1365-2044.2011.06989.x.

19. Hart RH, Vote BJ, Borthwick JH, McGeorge AJ, Worsley DR. Loss of vision caused by expansion of intraocular perfluoropropane (C(3)F(8)) gas during nitrous oxide anesthesia. Am J Ophthalmol. 2002;134(5):761–3. https://doi.org/10.1016/s0002-9394(02)01654-9.

20. Yang YF, Herbert L, Rüschen H, Cooling RJ. Nitrous oxide anaesthesia in the presence of intraocular gas can cause irreversible blindness. BMJ. 2002;325(7363):532–3. https://doi.org/10.1136/bmj.325.7363.532.

21. American Academy of Ophthalmology. "Surgical Treatment of Retinal Detachment. https://www.aao.org/disease-review/surgical-treatment-in-pediatric-retinal-detachment.

22. Connolly SE, Gordon KB, Horton JC. Salvage of vision after hypotension-induced ischemic optic neuropathy. Am J Ophthalmol. 1994;117(2):235–42. https://doi.org/10.1016/s0002-9394(14)73082-x.

23. Kim JY, Kim KN, Kim WJ, Lee YH. Acute bilateral visual loss related to orthostatic hypotension. Korean J Ophthalmol. 2013;27(5):372–5. https://doi.org/10.3341/kjo.2013.27.5.372.

24. American Academy of Ophthalmology. What is a Subconjunctival hemorrhage? https://www.aao.org/eye-health/diseases/what-is-subconjunctival-hemorrhage.

25. Jeong CH, Yoon S, Chung SW, Kim JY, Park KH, Huh JK. Subcutaneous emphysema related to dental procedures. J Korean Assoc Oral Maxillofac Surg. 2018;44(5):212–9. https://doi.org/10.5125/jkaoms.2018.44.5.212.

26. Fleischman D, Davis RM, Lee LB. Subcutaneous and periorbital emphysema following dental procedure. Ophthalmic Plast Reconstr Surg. 2014;30(2):e43–5. https://doi.org/10.1097/IOP.0b013e318295f982.

27. Tan S, Nikolarakos D. Subcutaneous emphysema secondary to dental extraction: a case report. Aust Dent J. 2017;62(1):95–7. https://doi.org/10.1111/adj.12464.

28. Lamont M, Booth A. Post-traumatic endophthalmitis following penetrating injury with dental needle. Eye. 2006;20:981–2. https://doi.org/10.1038/sj.eye.6702096.

29. Subramanian ML, Topping TM. Endogenous endophthalmitis after routine dental cleaning. Arch Ophthalmol. 2003;121(4):576–7. https://doi.org/10.1001/archopht.121.4.576.

Ear Exam for the Non-ENT

5

Daniel Choo

5.1 External Ear

5.1.1 Anatomy

The external ear consists of the auricle and external ear canal. Embryologically, the auricle arises from the first and second branchial arches and ascends during gestation from the mandible to its adult location. The external canal is primarily cartilaginous at birth, and the middle two thirds will ossify during childhood. Hair follicles and cerumen-producing glands are found in the skin of the cartilaginous portion.

The external ear structures include the helix which is the most superior rim of cartilaginous framework. The antihelix is just below this and superiorly separates to form the superior and inferior crus. The fossa triangularis is the flat space between the superior and the inferior crus. The conchal bowl is the largest indention that leads into the external ear canal. Additionally, the tragus is anterior to the opening of the external canal. The temporal bone also makes up the glenoid fossa which accepts the condylar process of the mandible to form the temporal mandibular joint (TMJ).

5.1.2 Exam

The external ear can be examined with careful inspection and palpation. The majority of the external ear canal and tympanic membrane are best examined with an otoscope.

D. Choo (✉)
Cincinnati Children's Pediatric Otolaryngology Head and Neck Surgery,
Cincinnati, OH, USA
e-mail: Daniel.choo@cchmc.org

S. Thikkurissy, S. Golkari (eds.), *History and Physical for the Pediatric Dental Patient*, https://doi.org/10.1007/978-3-031-51458-6_5

5.1.3 Pathology

5.1.3.1 Otitis Externa

Acute external otitis is common and frequently referred to as "swimmer's ear." This results from a diffuse infection of the external ear canal and occasionally nearby structures such as the ear cartilage and surrounding skin. The infection is usually preceded by localized trauma under warm, humid conditions. Symptoms include swelling and redness of the external canal, purulent drainage, and pain with manipulation of the external ear. This can be treated in most cases with topical antibiotic and steroid drops and occasionally oral antibiotics if severe.

Chronic otitis externa may also develop and, like other areas of the skin, may be due to eczematous changes. This can be treated with topical steroids.

5.1.3.2 Cerumen Impaction

Cerumen, or ear wax, is a common finding in the external ear canal. The ears are typically "self-cleaning," and wax can be removed by gently wiping the outside of the ear. If cerumen becomes pushed to the non-hair-bearing medial canal, an impaction may occur. This may need to be removed with instrumentation and can cause discomfort and conductive hearing loss.

5.1.3.3 TMJ Dysfunction

TMJ dysfunction is common and can manifest as ear pain. While more common in adult patients, children can also suffer from TMJ dysfunction related to joint inflammation. TMJ tenderness and popping and/or clicking with jaw opening can all be signs of TMJ dysfunction. These patients will often have a normal ear exam. Treatment can include joint rest and nonsteroidal anti-inflammatory drugs.

5.1.3.4 Odontogenic Referred Pain

Odontogenic referred pain, most commonly from the mandibular molars, can manifest as ear pain by way of the trigeminal nerve. Children who are teething can present with reports from parents of pulling at the ears. Like patients with TMJ dysfunction, the ear exam in these patients is often normal.

5.1.3.5 Microtia/Anotia/Ear Canal Stenosis/Atresia

Children with or without craniofacial differences can have irregularities of the external ear. This may include microtia or absence of the auricle, ear canal stenosis, or atresia. Microtia can be variable ranging from an overall small external ear to a complete absence of the pinna. Ear canal stenosis and atresia similarly may be a spectrum of a slightly narrowed canal to complete absence.

In the case of severe ear canal stenosis and canal atresia, there will be a conductive hearing loss, requiring amplification and possibly surgery.

5.1.3.6 Preauricular Anomalies

Preauricular pits or sinuses are small depressions most often found in the preauricular area just in front of the helix. These are common though occasionally can be associated with other findings or genetic syndromes. Hearing assessment is recommended. Excision of these may be pursued if there are issues with recurrent issues with infections or drainage of squamous debris.

5.2 Tympanic Membrane/Middle Ear

5.2.1 Anatomy

The middle ear is made up of the tympanic membrane, two muscles, and three ossicles. The eustachian tube additionally serves to aerate the middle ear space by connecting the middle ear to the nasopharynx. Embryologically, the middle ear is derived from the first and second pharyngeal arches. The main function of the middle ear is to conduct external sound to the inner ear structures.

5.2.2 Exam

The tympanic membrane is best seen with an otoscope. The tip of the otoscope is inserted into the external ear canal and gentle traction can be placed on the auricle. This allows for optimal viewing of the medial external ear canal and the tympanic membrane. The normal appearance of the membrane is translucent with a view into the aerated middle ear space. The tympanic membrane has normal surface landmarks including the malleus and the light reflex. Pneumatic otoscopy can provide additional information about the mobility of the tympanic membrane and the ventilation of the middle ear space.

5.2.3 Pathology

5.2.3.1 Otitis Media

Fluid within the middle ear, or otitis media, can give a dull appearance to the tympanic membrane. This will cause conductive hearing loss as the middle ear is unable to effectively transmit sound to the inner ear. Acutely infected fluid within the middle ear, or acute otitis media, can present with ear pain, irritability, and fever. In these cases, the tympanic membrane will often bulge with an angry erythematous appearance. Pain control and oral antibiotics are mainstays of treatment, while placement of pressure equalization tubes may be necessary in cases of prolonged middle ear fluid or recurrent acute otitis media.

5.2.3.2 Tympanic Membrane Perforation

Tympanic membrane perforations may result from infection, trauma, or iatrogenic causes such as prior ear tube placement. Perforations can vary in size and can cause conductive hearing loss. The treatment of these depends on the many factors, though surgical repair is an option.

5.2.3.3 Cholesteatoma

A cholesteatoma is an abnormal collection of skin cells that can either be congenital or develop as the result of long-standing ear disease. These can enlarge and over time erode the structures of the middle ear. Most cholesteatomas are the result of chronic ear disease and may present with prolonged ear drainage and conductive hearing loss. Surgery is the mainstay of treatment.

5.3   Inner Ear

5.3.1   Anatomy

The inner ear contains important structures for hearing and balance including the cochlea and the vestibular apparatus. The cochlea contains the organ of Corti which converts sound vibrations into electrical impulses. The vestibular apparatus, consisting of the semicircular canals and vestibule, relay position and movement of the head in space. The inner ear is derived from the otic placode and is the first structure of the ear to develop.

5.3.2   Exam

While the inner ear cannot be observed on physical exam, its function can be assessed through a variety of physical exam findings and objective tests.

5.3.3   Pathology

5.3.3.1 Vertigo

Dysfunction of the vestibular system results in vertigo which can be described as the sensation of rotation or motion when there is none. The most common cause of acute vertigo is calcium carbonate crystals settling with the semicircular canals known as benign paroxysmal positional vertigo. This can be treated with certain movements that help to move the crystals out of the semicircular canals. Other causes can be acute inflammation of the vestibular system, migraine related vertigo, or stroke.

5.3.3.2 Sensorineural Hearing Loss

Hearing loss from inner ear dysfunction is known as sensorineural hearing loss. This is the most common type of permanent hearing loss and can be treated with hearing amplification. Depending on the degree of hearing loss, cochlear implantation may be an option.

Assessment of the Lungs

6

Pravin Taneja

6.1 Introduction

Airway and respiratory complications are one of the most common causes of morbidity during sedation and general anesthesia in children. The goal of safe airway management is to anticipate and recognize respiratory compromise and to provide support of the airway in a timely manner during any sedation or anesthesia. The pediatric patients have significant anatomical and physiological differences compared with adults. These differences have a huge impact on the techniques and tools that the proceduralist or the anesthesia providers might choose to provide safe and effective control of the airway.

The airway in a pediatric patient continuously changes in size, shape, and position throughout its development from the neonate to the adult. Failure to assess and identify predictable difficulty in airway management and the failure to incorporate these findings into a treatment protocol can lead to a poor outcome. This review outlines the importance of airway assessment and discusses various methods of examination of the respiratory system. These would further help to identify a difficult airway in the subset of pediatric patients and plan appropriately for their procedural sedation.

The most important feature of conducting a safe pediatric sedation or anesthetic is the ability to assess and manage the pediatric airway. The assessment of the pediatric airway involves a detailed evaluation and examination of the upper airway and the respiratory system prior to any surgical or procedural intervention on any child. This assessment is imperative as airway and respiratory complications are among the most common causes of hypoxia during the perioperative critical incidents in pediatric anesthesia [1]. Furthermore, the incidence of these critical events in infants less than 1 year of age is four times more common than

P. Taneja (✉)
Temple University, Philadelphia, PA, USA
e-mail: Pravin.Taneja@towerhealth.org

in older children [2, 3]. Surgical procedures of the ear, nose, and throat pathology, eye surgery, oral surgery, and dental rehabilitations procedures are among the most frequent procedures requiring anesthesia and sedation in children. Their proximity to that of the airway makes them especially vulnerable to complications during the perioperative period.

6.2 Differences Between the Pediatric and Adult Airway

The respiratory system is structurally divided into the upper and lower respiratory airways. The upper airways extend from the external nares to the junction of the larynx with the trachea. This includes the nose, nasal cavity and the paranasal sinuses, the pharynx, and the larynx [4]. The lower airways comprise of the distal larynx, trachea, bronchial tree, and the lungs.

The upper airway parts of the respiratory tract allow the passage of air into the lungs. When we inhale, negative pressure in the thoracic cavity causes air and therefore oxygen to enter through the upper airway via the pharynx into the trachea to reach the alveoli. Subsequent gas exchange occurs between the alveoli and the blood stream providing oxygenation to the blood via the blood gas membrane [3].

There are important differences that occur continuously during its development, and the airway changes in size, shape, and position throughout its development from the neonate to the adult shape and structure [5]. Predictably, these differences are most pronounced at birth and in infants under 1 year of age. These differences in the infant's airway become more pronounced and recognizable as the child grows, and the upper airway assumes the characteristics of the adult airway by approximately 8 years of age. Thus, we can expect to see a progressive varied airway anatomy at different stages of development from birth to adulthood. Special attention needs to be devoted to the airway in infants and small children as they present with very different subset of challenges than older children and young adults. Apart from the obvious smaller size, there are other important anatomical and physiological factors that make it even more difficult and must be taken into consideration during their airway management (Fig. 6.1). This is especially important when they are under procedural sedation or unconscious under general anesthesia. Some of these factors and differences are summarized in Table 6.1.

The first anatomical difference between the pediatric and adult patient is that the head of a pediatric patient is larger relative to their body size, with a prominent occiput, leading to hyperflexion of the neck on the chest. This predisposes them to airway obstruction during sleep as the neck is in flexed when they lie supine on a flat surface. A neck or shoulder roll can generally facilitate to counter this flexion and relieve the airway obstruction.

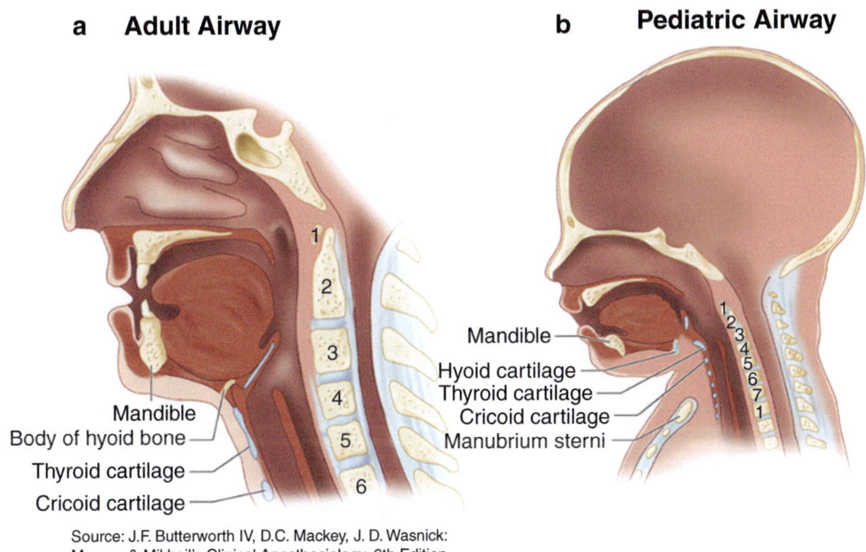

Fig. 6.1 Diagrammatic description of the sagittal section of the adult (**a**) and infant (**b**) airway depicting the differences between the adult (**a**) and the pediatric airway (**b**). (Reproduced with permission from Publisher of Adapted from the Clinical Anatomy for Anesthesiologists @ New York, NY: Appleton & Lange; 1988)

Table 6.1 Anatomical differences between the pediatric and adult airway

Differences between the pediatric and adult airway
• Smaller dimensions
• Head relatively larger in infants
• Neck is shorter than adults
• Tongue relatively larger
• Large lingual tonsils
• Prominent buccal fat
• Narrow nasal passage
• Smaller jaw
• Longer palate
• Long and elongated epiglottis
(a) Larynx located more cephalad (C4)
• Vocal cords angled more anteriorly
• Airway narrowest at the cricoid cartilage
• Trachea is shorter and narrower
• Decreased muscle tone
• Soft and reactive airway in infants and children
• Ribs are almost horizontal
• Weaker intercostal and diaphragmatic muscles

6.3   Assessment of the Airway

Assessment and the management of a pediatric airway is always a great challenge. The pediatric patients have significant anatomical and physiological differences compared with adults. The pediatric airway is substantially different from the adult airway and minimal obstruction leads to a rapid desaturation in infants and small children. The lack of a patent airway or breathing adequacy is the most common reason for development of hypoxia.

In order to safely perform the management of any airway, it is essential for the providers and clinicians to have a thorough knowledge of the important anatomical and physiological features related to the airway as well as knowledge of the various tools and equipment that are available for this purpose. Knowledge of the developmental and functional anatomy of the airway in children forms the basis of understanding the pathological conditions that may present in the patients. These collective understanding in turn allows for a comprehensive assessment of the pediatric airway to take place, including a detailed medical history, a thorough clinical examination, and necessary specific investigative procedures.

6.4   Oral Cavity

The tongue in small children is large relative to the size of the oral cavity, and the mandible is shorter. This large tongue easily apposes on to the palate and blocks the pharynx leading to an upper airway obstruction. These represent one of the most common causes of airway obstruction and desaturation in sedated and/or unconscious infants and children. The large tongue and the presence of buccal fat in many infants and children are not uncommon which can further reduce the space in the mouth cavity. Collectively, these may also hamper attempts to visualize the back of the mouth or the glottis during examination or laryngoscopy. This upper airway obstruction can many a times be overcome by either a jaw-thrust maneuver which will help lift the tongue and relieve the obstruction or depress the tongue with the placement and use of an oropharyngeal airway device.

The oropharynx extends from the soft palate to the tip of the epiglottis. At the entrance to the oropharynx is a collection of lymphoid tissue known as Waldeyer's ring. This consists of the lingual tonsil at the base of the tongue and bilateral palatine tonsils. The nasopharyngeal and tubal tonsils also form part of this ring. Inflammation of these lymphoid tissues may obstruct breathing efforts in conscious patients and may make laryngoscopy difficult because of an increase in size of the tissue or associated masseter spasm [6].

6.5   Nasal Cavity

The external nose is made up of the nasal bones, the nasal part of the frontal bones, and the frontal processes of the maxillae. The nasal cavity is subdivided by the nasal septum into two separate compartments that open to the exterior via the nares and into the nasopharynx via the choanae or posterior nasal apertures [7]. Immediately within the nares lies the vestibule, which contains an area of arterial anastomosis known as Little's area. Epistaxis most commonly occurs from this zone. Application of pressure at this area is essential to achieve hemostasis to stop the epistaxis.

During development, the nose and the nasal cavities extend under the influence of the posteriorly directed fusion of the palatal processes. These changes cause the membrane that separates the palatal processes from the oral cavity to become progressively thinner and eventually rupture to form the choanae or posterior nasal apertures [5]. Failure of this membrane to rupture or open results in a nasal obstruction known as "choanal atresia." Depending on the unruptured membrane, this obstruction could be either unilateral or bilateral. Severity of presenting symptoms of difficulty in breathing would be determined by the significance of the blockage.

In addition, the nose and nasal cavity in younger children have more mucosa and larger lymphoid tissue than in older children and adults leading to increased resistance to airflow through the nasal passages [7]. Prominent adenoids and tonsils are frequently found in preschool age children and are a common reason to present for elective surgeries. All these factors contribute to the loss of upper airway space which can lead to difficulty with mask ventilation, obstruction during spontaneous ventilation, and can make laryngoscopy more difficult. In addition, sedatives, hypnotic, and anesthetic drugs cause a loss of tone of upper airway muscles which further result in potential upper airway obstruction [8].

Furthermore, in children the already smaller and narrower nasal passages get readily blocked by mucous and secretions from the commonly occurring upper respiratory infections, edema, or blood. Nasal obstruction can cause serious problems, especially in infants as neonates and young infants are "obligate nose breathers," until 6 months of age, and they may not immediately be able to switch to mouth breathing. Such conditions may increase the work of breathing or cause desaturation and similarly contribute to difficulties with management of the airway under sedation or general anesthesia.

6.6   Epiglottis and Larynx

The epiglottis in infants and young children is more "U" shaped compared to the flat-shaped epiglottis in adults. Further, in children the epiglottis is characteristically relatively short and stubby and is angled posteriorly at an angle of 45° above the glottis and away from the long axis of the trachea. This position makes it difficult to control via vallecular suspension with a curved laryngoscope blade during intubation. To overcome this feature, a straight laryngoscope blade is preferable to a curved laryngoscope blade in this situation [9].

The larynx is situated between the pharynx and the trachea, extending from the base of the tongue to the cricoid cartilage. It is the structure of phonation in humans and protects the tracheobronchial tree during swallowing and coughing [9]. The larynx consists of the thyroid cartilage, the cricoid cartilage, a paired arytenoid, and the epiglottis, along with the small corniculate and cuneiform cartilages. Of these structures the thyroid cartilage is the largest and anteriorly it forms the laryngeal prominence, commonly known as the Adam's apple [6].

The larynx is situated relatively higher in the neck in infants and children. At birth, the lower border of the cricoid cartilage lies opposite the lower border of the C4 vertebra. At age of 6 years, it is at the level of the C5 vertebra, whereas it lies at the level of the C6 vertebra in adults [7]. This cephalad position of the infant's larynx effectively creates a more of an acute angle between the base of the tongue and the glottic opening (Fig. 6.1). This makes the glottic opening appear anterior which makes visualization of the cords very difficult during direct laryngoscopy. Furthermore, because of the small size of the cricoid cartilage in children, and the fact that it is a complete ring, the presence of mucosal edema at this site from any causative factors will severely compromise the airway.

6.7 Vocal Cords and Trachea

The adult vocal cords lie perpendicular to the laryngeal axis, whereas the infant's vocal cords are angled in an anterocaudal position. In this the anterior attachment of the vocal cord is at a more inferior level than the posterior attachment, thus making it not only a little more difficult to view the vocal cords but making the insertion of the endotracheal tube more challenging and traumatic. The narrowest portion of the adult airway is at the level of the vocal cords itself, whereas the narrowest portion of the pediatric airway is located below the level of the vocal cords at the cricoid cartilage. This unique feature gives the pediatric airway its "funnel shape" as opposed to the "cylindrical shape" of the adult airway (Fig. 6.1). At this level the mucosa of the vocal cords is lined with pseudostratified ciliated epithelium that is loosely bound to the underlying areolar tissue. Any trauma to these tissues results in edema, and even a little circumferential edema significantly encroaches on the small area of the infant airway. This reduces the lumen and greatly increases the resistance to flow, causing stridor. Insertion of an endotracheal tube similarly encroaches on the space as the internal diameter of the tube essentially becomes the area for gas flow and further increases the airway resistance. This becomes more significant with smaller infants.

6.8 Ribs and Lungs

Infant and young pediatric patients have immature laryngeal, tracheal, and bronchial structures. The trachea is relatively short in length (approximately 5 cm in the neonate), so precise placement and fixation of the endotracheal tube are essential.

The pediatric airway is highly compliant, and the cartilaginous support is less developed than in the adult airway. The bronchioles, alveoli, and lungs are also not fully developed. The alveoli fully mature to the adult level and function by about 8 years of age.

The ribs in younger infant and neonates are soft, cartilaginous, and almost horizontally situated. They have poorly developed intercostal muscles, and their chest walls are more compliant than in adults. Thus, the children rely heavily on their diaphragm for their ventilation [10]. The abdominal viscera in infants and toddlers are bulky and can hinder diaphragmatic excursion, especially if the gastrointestinal tract is distended.

The elastic nature of these airway structures makes them particularly susceptible to mechanical compression, stretching, and distortion by internal or external pressure differences. The tracheal cartilages are soft and can easily be compressed by the fingers. This can lead to increased susceptibility of dynamic airway collapse in the presence of any airway obstruction [11]. Due to this compressibility and susceptibility to external compression, extreme care needs to be taken when holding a face mask on the face and neck of these smaller patients. Improper pressure on the chin and neck can lead to near total airway obstruction from compression of the larynx. Studies have also demonstrated that airway obstruction during general anesthesia is related to a reduction in laryngeal muscle tone. Loss of muscle tone in the pharynx leads to airway obstruction at the level of the soft palate and epiglottis [11].

6.9 Preoperative Airway Assessment

The pediatric airway poses a challenge particularly for those who do not anesthetize or sedate small children on a regular basis. Evaluation of the airway is an integral part of preoperative assessment for every child who undergoes procedural sedation or anesthesia. Assessment of the pediatric airway is often difficult because the child is frequently unable to cooperate with the evaluation. The assessment of the lung involves a thorough evaluation and review of the airway and the respiratory system. Primary care providers can play a significant role in creating a safe perioperative environment by providing an accurate assessment of the child's current medical condition and by working to optimize the child's clinical status in preparation for surgery, thus minimizing the risk to the patient in the perioperative period. A comprehensive method for assessment of the pediatric airway begins with a detailed medical history and a thorough clinical examination both of which are facilitated by knowledge of the normal anatomy. In contrast to adults, most children with difficult airways are recognized before induction of anesthesia, but problems may arise in all children.

Questions during the medical history should be directed toward eliciting indications of anything suggesting a potentially difficult airway during the planned procedure. These questions should include any history of previous respiratory illness or a history of any injuries or surgical procedures involving the airway. Details should be noted of any complications that occurred during previous anesthesia, particularly those related to the airway. A history of cessation of breathing or excessive daytime somnolence is suggestive of obstructive sleep apnea. Questions such as a history of snoring, daytime drowsiness, or stopping breathing during sleep may help to identify children with obstructive sleep apnea syndrome (OSAS).

Specific questions should also be asked about the child's respiration, feeding habits, speech, as well as the presence and nature of any cough. Further questions should probe and elucidate any history of current or recent symptoms suggesting upper respiratory infection (URI), difficulty in speaking, difficulty breathing, difficulty feeding, hoarseness, noisy breathing, or coughing.

6.10   Airway Examination

The examination of any airway is necessary before any procedural sedation or anesthesia intervention. The recommendation is to be able to predict a difficult airway in any patient and be able to anticipate and prepare for any such circumstances. Some of these predictive factors that would indicate for a difficult or challenging airway management are listed in Table 6.2. These would give the providers time to prepare and gather the necessary equipment needed for any such needed intervention.

The airway examination begins with a thorough examination of the head and neck areas, and much information can be gathered from the general appearance of the child, with special reference to obstructive sleep apnea syndrome (OSAS), body mass index (BMI), and characteristics of the face. Kohler et al. studied that obesity is a significant predictor of upper airway obstruction in children who snore during their sleep. He also found that the association of body mass index with upper airway obstruction is much stronger among African American children [12]. A detailed exam and characteristic features of the mouth and the face should be documented. This should be followed by a careful examination of the chest and the lungs for disorders of respiration.

Table 6.2 Features suggestive of a difficult pediatric airway during an examination

Features suggestive of a difficult airway in children
• Obesity/OSA
• Limited mouth opening
(b) High arched or narrow palate
• Small mandible (micrognathia)
• Overbite (long upper incisor teeth)
• Long upper incisor teeth
• Large tongue (macroglossia)
• Narrow submandibular space
• Decreased thyromental distance
• Short length neck
• Increased neck circumference
• Limited neck and head mobility
(c) Edema, vomit, or blood in the airway
• Syndromic facial features

Many physical exam findings which are well-known to predict and indicate a potential difficult airway in adults are also applicable to children. Limited head extension, reduced mandibular space, and increased tongue thickness have been shown to be the most reliable predictors of difficult airway intubation [13]. Thus, in the absence of any obvious area of abnormality or any specific congenital syndrome associated with a difficult airway, most difficult airways can be recognized by performing the following three basic evaluations:

1. Oropharyngeal and nasopharyngeal examination
2. Assessment of the atlanto-occipital joint mobility
3. Assessment of the potential displacement area

The examination of these areas correctly predicts a difficult airway in adults virtually all of the time. The applicability of these tests may not be 100% in pediatric patients as many of them require patient cooperation. Participation of children in any tests is always unpredictable and very challenging.

6.11 Oropharyngeal and Nasopharyngeal Examination

This involves a close observation of the child followed by examination of the mouth and nose areas. An evaluation of the symmetry of head, face, ears, cheeks, and neck is crucial as asymmetry is found in many syndromic cases. The degree of mouth opening, presence or absence of oral pathology, and oral hygiene should be noted. The relative size of the oral cavity and mouth opening is assessed by asking the child to open his or her mouth. To adequately judge the mouth opening, use the child's own fingers for measurements. The distance between upper and lower incisors with full mouth opening normally should be a minimum of two finger breadths or more. Any less of a mouth opening is indicative of a potential difficult airway. A close attention to loose teeth in children is important as they may break and get lodged in the airway with disastrous consequences. Further, the length of the incisor teeth should also be inspected as the longer incisors represent a possible difficult airway as less space becomes available in the mouth for laryngoscopy and endotracheal tube. The inter-incisor distance can also be assessed at this time, where in an inter-incisor distance less than two patients' own finger breadths have been associated with a difficult airway. The child's facial expression or the presence of nasal flaring may suggest respiratory distress. Mouth-breathing or drooling often occur in the presence of enlarged tonsils or adenoids. The patency of the nasal apertures should be assessed, as well as the amount, nature, and color of any nasal discharge. The tongue, teeth, pharynx, and palate should be inspected for abnormalities. Examination of the child's mucous membranes of the mouth may detect cyanosis secondary to hypoxemia.

The Mallampati classification system as modified by Samsoon and Young classifies the degree of airway difficulty based on the ability to visualize the faucial pillars, soft palate, and uvula during an oral examination. The Mallampati classification

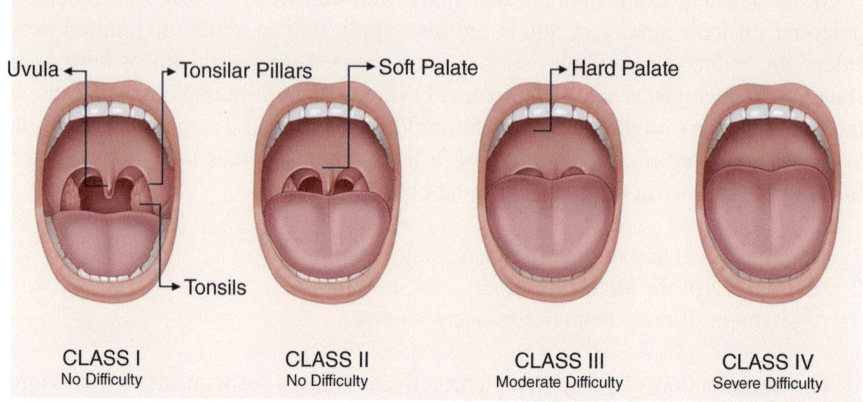

Fig. 6.2 Mallampati classification as a predictor of difficult intubation

Table 6.3 Modified Mallampati score for airway assessment

Mallampati grade	Visual oral anatomic view	Predictive value
Class I	Complete visualization of the soft palate, tonsillar pillars, and the uvula	No difficulty
Class II	Complete visualization of the soft palate with partial view of the tonsillar pillars and the uvula	No difficulty
Class III	Visualization of only the base of the uvula and the soft palate. No view of the tonsillar pillars and the distal uvula	Moderate difficulty
Class IV	No visualization of the soft palate, tonsillar pillars, or the uvula	Severe difficulty

Adapted from the article of Samsoon and Young (Anaesthesia, 1987;42:487–90) [15]

scale is a pictorial grade scale (Fig. 6.2) that was created to predict difficult intubation before general anesthesia [14, 15] and is now routinely used for this purpose in operating rooms worldwide [16]. It is very informative and one of the easiest exams to do by the bedside of the patient. The patient should be sitting upright with their head in a neutral position. Ask the patient to open their mouth and extend their tongue. The observer looks to see if structures can clearly be visualized in the back of the throat (Table 6.3).

This tool grades the level of difficulty that could be expected during laryngoscopy and intubation based upon the examination finding of the oral cavity. Over the period of subsequent years, this tool has been modified for use in predicting various airway evaluation parameters like difficult preoperative laryngoscopy, intubation, and difficult bag-valve-mask ventilation. These predictive parameters have further been extrapolated and applied to patients outside of the operating rooms undergoing procedural sedation. This applicability and utility of the Mallampati classification scale has made it a widely recommended tool as a routine screening element even before procedural sedations. The American Academy of Pediatrics (AAP) recommends the routine use of the Mallampati classification for airway evaluation prior to any routine pre-sedation health assessment in all areas of care including the dental procedures, radiology suites, gastrointestinal endoscopy suites, and the emergency department [16–18].

The Mallampati score is intended to supplement, but not replace, the baseline clinical judgment of a general multidimensional airway evaluation. Although popular and used widely, there have been many questions regarding the accuracy, reliability, and feasibility of the Mallampati score especially toward its use in the management before procedural sedations. Its use and utility in infants and young children have also been questioned.

There have been many studies in children corroborating the validity of this predictive scale. It is important to note that the Mallampati score is intended to supplement, but not replace, the baseline clinical judgment of a general multidimensional airway evaluation. It is also crucial to recognize and acknowledge that the quality and reliability of the general airway evaluation is at times hindered or limited by emergency situations, uncooperative patients, and unavailable medical history. Additionally, a cooperative patient is required to open the mouth and protrude the tongue, and so the Mallampati assessment can be impossible for patients who cannot or will not comply. However, children may not cooperate for a proper oral airway exam, and an isolated class 3 or 4 score in an uncooperative child with otherwise normal airway exam may not indicate a potential difficult airway.

6.12 Assessment of the Atlanto-Occipital Joint Mobility

This assessment evaluates the mobility and the range of movement of the head and neck region. Normal mouth opening, mandibular size, and neck mobility are fundamental to the success of intubation using the most common technique, direct laryngoscopy. Flexion, extension, and lateral rotation movements of the head and neck should be evaluated and documented. Extension of the head with upper cervical spine mobility assists in opening the airway during sedation procedures. Any decrease in the range of movement at the atlanto-occipital joint leads to the poor visualization of the pharynx and the glottis area during oral examination and subsequent laryngoscopy, respectively. This would lead to a difficulty in intubation and maintaining oxygenation during spontaneous ventilation. Examination of the neck may also reveal other deformities of the cervical spine or cervical lymphadenopathy. These may most commonly indicate signs of existing infection or be a precursor to a malignancy which should be further investigated.

6.13 Examination of the Chest and Lungs

This includes the examination of the lower part of the airway which includes the trachea, bronchioles, lungs, and chest wall. Begin the examination by listening to the child's voice or cry as hoarseness or a weak cry may occur in the presence of airway obstruction at the level of the vocal cords. Observe the work of breathing if

Table 6.4 Normal respiratory rate in children

Normal respiratory rate in children		
Age group		Respiratory rate (breaths/minute)
Infants	<1 year	30–57
Toddler	1–3 years	22–46
Preschooler	3–6 years	20–29
School-age	6–12 years	16–24
Adolescents	13–18 years	13–21
Adults	>18 years	12–16

the child is breathing heavy or making noises during respiration. Stridor is a high-pitched sound that is indicative of laryngeal or tracheal obstruction. Inspiratory stridor suggests obstruction at or above the upper trachea, and expiratory stridor suggests obstruction of the lower trachea or bronchi. Excessive flaccidity of the soft epiglottis and the loose aryepiglottic folds can cause these structures to collapse on inspiration, resulting in stridor. Continue next to evaluate the respiratory rate.

6.13.1 Respiratory Rate

Assess the child's respiratory rate for 60 s to calculate the number of breaths per minute. Note any asymmetries in the expiratory and inspiratory phases of respiration as the expiratory phase is often prolonged in conditions of asthma exacerbations. The range of a normal respiratory rate varies significantly depending on the age of the child, and this should be considered. The normal respiratory rate for different age groups is listed in Table 6.4.

When observing the respiratory pattern and rate, assess for signs of increased work of breathing which include difficulty speaking or feeding and expiratory grunting. Both these suggest underlying respiratory pathology that would need further investigation prior to any elective sedation or anesthesia for any procedures.

6.14 Chest and Lungs

The shape of the chest should be observed for the frequency and depth of each breath during respiration. Chest hyper-expansion also known as barrel chest can be associated with asthma and chronic respiratory obstruction. The presence of Harrison's sulcus, which is the indrawing of the chest wall from long-term diaphragmatic tug, has been found to be associated with poorly controlled asthma.

Further inspection of the respiratory system can reveal the degree of the chest expansion, symmetry of the chest expansions, and the presence of any chest wall recession or retractions. Asymmetric movement of the chest wall may indicate underlying pneumothorax or consolidation. Conditions of the chest wall where the chest has a caved-in or sunken appearance of the chest is known as pectus excavatum and is seen in many connective tissue disorders like the Marfan syndrome.

Pectus carinatum is a condition where there is protrusion of the sternum and ribs as seen in genetic disorders like Noonan syndrome. Most of these conditions have other organs involved and should be investigated thoroughly prior to any elective surgical procedures. Additionally, signs of chest wall recession such as supraclavicular, intercostal, or subcostal muscle recession are also indicative of ominous intrathoracic pathology that should be investigated.

Evidence of use of accessory muscles of respiration can be inferred from the presence of nasal flaring, abdominal breathing, or head bobbing secondary to sternocleidomastoid contractions. These signs are seen during labored breathing and are one of the earliest signs of airway obstruction. The use of accessory muscles also indicates underlying severe disease and respiratory distress and further signifies that the forced expiratory volume in 1 s (FEV1) is decreased to 30% of the normal or less.

Auscultation of the lungs has an important place in the diagnosis of certain respiratory diseases such as bronchial asthma or pneumonia. Children have thinner chest walls than adults and therefore louder breath sounds. A child's chest has cartilaginous structures that increase lung compliance and promotes cooperation during auscultation [19]. When auscultating the chest, it is important to have a systematic approach that allows to compare each area on both the right and the left as you progress. Assess the quality and volume of breath sounds and note any added sounds like rales, rhonchi, stridor, or wheezing.

6.15 Possible Complications

6.15.1 Cough

Cough is a common presenting symptom of respiratory abnormality and is often associated with upper respiratory tract infection. Other common causes of cough in children are asthma, gastroesophageal reflux disease (GERD), bronchitis, and environmental tobacco smoke exposure. Between 35 and 40% of school-age children still cough 10 days after the onset of a common cold, and 10% of preschool children have cough 25 days after respiratory tract infection [20]. It may be caused by stimuli arising in the mucosa of any part of the respiratory tract. In children, cough can be distressing and has a major impact on a child's sleep, school, and ability to play.

To diagnose the etiology of the cough, we need to know regarding the frequency, severity, and character of the cough. Other factors including the situation and nature of the lesion responsible for the cough, the presence or absence of sputum, and the presence of coexisting abnormalities such as impairment of ventilatory function need to be reviewed. In acute respiratory tract infection, the cough is usually productive and associated with purulent nasal secretions. Resolution of cough is spontaneous in most children [21]. A list of different types of cough with possible diagnosis is presented in Table 6.5.

Table 6.5 Common recognizable cough characteristics in children [22]

Cough type	Suggested underlying process
Cough with wheeze	Asthma, viral-induced wheeze, subglottic stenosis
Barking or brassy cough	Croup, laryngomalacia, tracheomalacia
Dry cough	Allergies, tuberculosis
Paroxysmal (with or without inspiratory "whoop")	Pertussis and para-pertussis
Chronic wet cough in mornings only	Suppurative lung disease, sinusitis

Table 6.6 Congenital syndromes with features associated with potential difficult airway

Syndromes with potential difficult airway management
• Pierre Robin syndrome
• Treacher Collins syndrome
• Mucopolysaccharidoses (Hunter's and Hurler's syndrome)
• Choanal atresia (CHARGE syndrome)
• Apert syndrome
• Beckwith-Wiedemann syndrome
• Crouzon syndrome
Freeman-Sheldon syndrome
• Down syndrome
• Goldenhar syndrome
• Klippel-Feil sequence

6.15.1.1 Congenital Syndromes

Many congenital syndromes are associated with potentially difficult airway management, and these add an additional layer of complexity in the management of these patients. Syndromes with face malformations, especially those with a short mandible and ear deformity, should alert the anesthesiologist and the care providers as these are often associated with difficult airways [6]. Some of the more commonly encountered congenital syndromes with potential airway complications are summarized in Table 6.6. Detailed description of individual syndromes and their significant features is beyond the scope of this review, but a difficult airway is the common link in all of the listed syndromes. Any of these syndromes should raise red flags and concerns with every clinician and anesthesia providers. Further, all the decisions to provide anesthesia or any procedural sedation in children with congenital syndromes should be absolutely deliberate, methodical, and carefully evaluated. It is highly recommended that these children get their procedural intervention performed at care facilities equipped to take care of the challenges and complications that may arise from a difficult airway intervention.

6.16 Conclusion

Pediatric airway management has its unique sets of challenges. Strict adherence to safe and simple principles can affect the confidence and outcome in these patients. It is essential to pay attention to the details and do the due diligence in preoperative and preprocedural assessment including a comprehensive history and a thorough clinical examination. Knowledge of functional airway anatomy is invaluable for an understanding of the pathological airway conditions that present within the pediatric population. Use the predictive value of the assessment tools to make appropriate and rational decisions which may complicate general anesthesia. Be careful of pediatric patients with upper respiratory infections and with "just a cold" and patients with congenital syndromes. Unlike adults, most difficult airway patients can be identified prior to the procedural intervention. It is important to remember that no ideal method of assessment exists, and unanticipated difficulty will still occur from time to time.

References

1. Morray JP, Geiduschek JM, Ramamoorthy C, Haberkern CM, Hackel A, Caplan RA, et al. Anesthesia-related cardiac arrest in children: initial findings of the pediatric perioperative cardiac arrest (POCA) registry. Anesthesiology. 2000;93(1):6–14.
2. Murat I, Constant I, Maud'huy H. Perioperative anaesthetic morbidity in children: a database of 24,165 anaesthetics over a 30-month period. Paediatr Anaesth. 2004;14(2):158–66.
3. Tay CL, Tan GM, Ng SB. Critical incidents in paediatric anaesthesia: an audit of 10,000 anaesthetics in Singapore. Paediatr Anaesth. 2001;11(6):711–8.
4. Westmore RF, Muntz HR, McGill TJI. Pediatric otolaryngology, principles and practice pathways. New York: Thieme Medical Publishers; 2000.
5. Holzman R. Anatomy and embryology of the paediatric airway. Anesthesiol Clin N Am. 1998;16:707–27.
6. Roberts JT. Clinical management of the airway. Philadelphia: W. B. Saunders Company; 1994.
7. Dickison AE. The normal and abnormal pediatric airway. Recognition and management of obstruction. Clin Chest Med. 1987;8:583–96.
8. Sunder RA, Haile DT, Farrell PT, Sharma A. Pediatric airway management: current practices and future directions. Paediatr Anaesth. 2012;22(10):1008–15.
9. Wheeler DS, Spaeth JP, Mehta R, Hariprakash SP, Cox PN. Assessment and management of the pediatric airway. In: Resuscitation and stabilization of the critically ill child. London: Springer London; 2009. p. 1–30.
10. Saikia D, Mahanta B. Cardiovascular and respiratory physiology in children. Indian J Anaesth. 2019;63(9):690–7.
11. Nandi PR, Charlesworth CH, Taylor SJ, et al. The effect of general anesthesia on the pharynx. Br J Anaesth. 1991;66:157–62.
12. Kohler M, Lushington K, Couper R, Martin J, van den Heuvel C, Pamula Y, et al. Obesity and risk of sleep related upper airway obstruction in Caucasian children. J Clin Sleep Med. 2008;4(2):129–36.
13. Crawley SM, Dalton AJ. Predicting the difficult airway. BJA Educ. 2015;15(5):253–8.
14. Mallampati SR, Gatt SP, Gugino LD, Desai SP, Waraksa B, Freiberger D, et al. A clinical sign to predict difficult tracheal intubation: a prospective study. Can Anaesth Soc J. 1985;32(4):429–34.
15. Samsoon LT, Young G. Difficult tracheal intubation: a retrospective study. Anaesthesia. 1987;42(5):487–90.
16. Pediatrics CCJWSAA. American Academy of Pediatric Dentistry; AAP Guidelines for monitoring and management of pediatric patients before, during, and after sedation for diagnostic and therapeutic procedures: update 2016. Pediatrics. 2016;138.
17. Green SM, Roback MG. Is the Mallampati score useful for emergency department airway management or procedural sedation? Ann Emerg Med. 2019;74(2):251–9.
18. Olsen JW, Barger RL Jr, Doshi SK. Moderate sedation: what radiologists need to know. AJR Am J Roentgenol. 2013;201(5):941–6.

19. Dionne RA, Driscoll EJ, Gelfman SS, Sweet JB, Butler DP, Wirdzek PR. Cardiovascular and respiratory response to intravenous diazepam, fentanyl, and methohexital in dental outpatients. J Oral Surg. 1981;39:343–9.
20. Hay AD. The duration of acute cough in pre-school children presenting to primary care: a prospective cohort study. Fam Pract. 2003;20(6):696–705.
21. Brooke AM, Lambert PC, Burton PR, Clarke C, Luyt DK, Simpson H. Recurrent cough: natural history and significance in infancy and early childhood. Pediatr Pulmonol. 1998;26(4):256–61.
22. Schaefer MK, Shehab N, Cohen AL, Budnitz DS. Adverse events from cough and cold medications in children. Pediatrics. 2008;121(4):783–7.

Assessment of the Heart

Cara J. Riley

Before treating a pediatric patient in the dental office, it is important to understand the status of the patient's cardiovascular system. Patients with cardiovascular disease may require modifications to treatment that can be determined in consultation with the patient's medical team. Furthermore, patients with moderate to severe cardiovascular disease typically are not good candidates for care under sedation in the dental office setting [1]. In order to ensure the correct triage of patients, it is essential that the dentist complete a basic cardiovascular examination [1]. While it is true that most cardiac lesions will declare themselves before a patient presents for dental treatment—indeed, the majority of children with serious congenital heart disease are diagnosed prenatally or during the neonatal period [2]—there exists the possibility that congenital heart disease or acquired heart disease will present beyond infancy. A thorough history and physical exam will extract evidence of such cardiovascular abnormalities. Many providers find assessment of the heart to be challenging and intimidating, especially the interpretation of heart sounds [1]. Following a systematic approach and considering findings from the entire examination can make the process more straightforward and fruitful. Being able to distinguish abnormal from normal and knowing when to refer for medical consultation are realistic goals and fundamental to patient safety.

Understanding cardiac anatomy and physiology is key to the successful assessment of the heart. The first part of this chapter will review cardiac anatomy, circulation, and the cardiac cycle. The rest of the chapter is dedicated to the process of examining the cardiovascular system.

C. J. Riley (✉)
Department of Anesthesiology, Children's Hospital Colorado, Aurora, CO, USA

© The Author(s), under exclusive license to Springer Nature Switzerland AG 2023
S. Thikkurissy, S. Golkari (eds.), *History and Physical for the Pediatric Dental Patient*, https://doi.org/10.1007/978-3-031-51458-6_7

44

7.1   Cardiac Anatomy

The anterior cardiac surface against the chest wall is occupied mostly by the right ventricle. The right ventricle and the pulmonary artery are found behind and to the left of the sternum. Where the right ventricle and pulmonary artery meet—at the second interspaces close to the sternum—is termed the base of the heart [3]. The interspace, or intercostal space, is the area between the ribs, and each space is numbered according to which rib is superior.

The left lateral margin of the heart is occupied by the left ventricle. The left ventricle is behind and to the left of the right ventricle. The tip of the left ventricle is called the cardiac apex, and it is here that the apical impulse can be palpated. In a normal heart, this is also known as the point of maximal impulse (PMI) [3]. The apical impulse represents the early pulsation of the left ventricle as it contracts and touches the chest wall. It is generally felt in the midclavicular line at the level of the xiphoid process. A normal apical impulse feels brisk and tapping. Apical impulses can be abnormal in terms of diameter, amplitude, and duration; if those things are increased, it is suspicious for left ventricular hypertrophy or volume overload of the left ventricle [3].

The right heart border is formed by the right atrium, while the left atrium is mostly posterior. The atria are not directly examinable.

The pulmonary artery, as previously mentioned, is found to the left of the sternum. It quickly bifurcates into left and right branches. The aorta emerges from the left ventricle, crossing posterior to the pulmonary artery, to be found to the right of the pulmonary artery before arching backward and down. To the right of the aorta, the superior vena cava empties into the right atrium. The inferior vena cava also empties into the right atrium, but from below. The venae cavae carry venous blood to the heart from the upper and lower portions of the body [3] (Fig. 7.1).

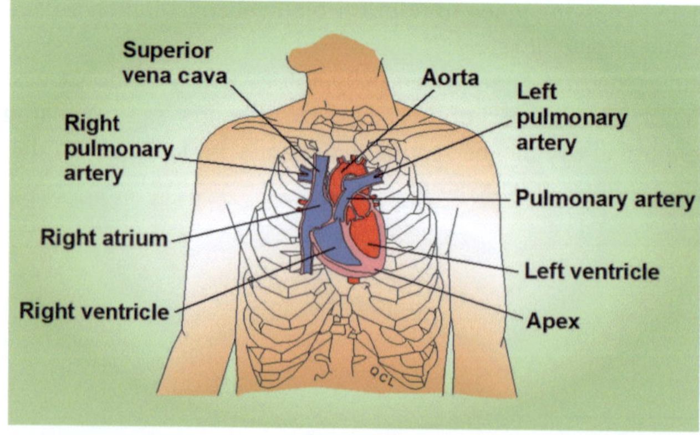

Fig. 7.1 Cardiac anatomy

7.2   Cardiac Circulation

Circulation through the heart begins with deoxygenated blood from the body returning to the right atrium via the venae cavae. The deoxygenated blood travels from the right atrium to the right ventricle, where it travels to the lungs via the pulmonary artery. The blood is oxygenated and returns to the heart via the pulmonary veins, which empty into the left atrium. This oxygenated blood then flows to the left ventricle, where it is pumped out to the body through the aorta. In between the atria and ventricles are the atrioventricular valves: the tricuspid on the right and the mitral on the left. In between the ventricles and the great vessels are the semilunar valves, known as the pulmonic and aortic valves. Heart sounds arise from the closing of valves (Fig. 7.2).

Heart valves can be affected by three primary pathologic conditions: regurgitation, stenosis, and prolapse. A regurgitant valve allows backflow into the proximal chamber when it closes, whereas a stenotic valve impedes forward flow into the distal chamber when it is open. Prolapse occurs when valve leaflets bulge into the proximal chamber upon closing of the valve. Regurgitation and stenosis typically cause a murmur, whereas prolapse may cause a click on auscultation. These three conditions do not only occur in isolation; they can occur together [4]. Valve disease in children is caused by congenital defects or inflammatory damage following rheumatic fever. Longstanding valve disease can lead to enlargement of the heart chambers and heart failure.

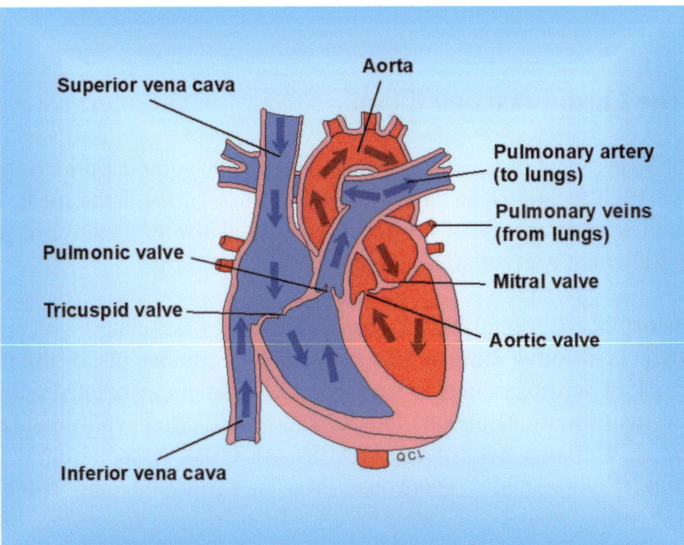

Fig. 7.2 Cardiac circulation

7.3 The Cardiac Cycle

Systole is the period of ventricular contraction, whereas diastole is the period of ventricular relaxation. During systole, the left and right ventricles contract and pressure rises until most of the blood has been ejected into the aorta and pulmonary artery, respectively. During diastole, the ventricles relax, ventricular pressure decreases, and blood flows from the atria into the ventricles. During systole, the atrioventricular (tricuspid and mitral) valves are closed to prevent regurgitation backward into the atria, whereas the semilunar (pulmonic and aortic valves) are open. In contrast, during diastole, the atrioventricular valves are open and the semilunar valves are closed.

Heart sounds are effectively caused by changes in pressure within the heart chambers, which in turn has an effect on the heart valves. The left ventricle creates a rapidly rising increase in pressure as it contracts. At the point that left ventricular pressure exceeds the pressure in the left atrium, the mitral valve closes. This produces the first heart sound, S1, and is the official start to systole. As the pressure in the left ventricle continues to rise, it quickly exceeds the pressure in the aorta, as well. This forces the aortic valve to open. Normally, maximal left ventricular pressure corresponds to systolic blood pressure [3]. Once most of the blood has been ejected from the ventricles, ventricular pressure begins to decrease. When the pressure in the ventricles drops below the pressure in their corresponding great vessel (aorta or pulmonary artery), the semilunar valves close. The closure of the aortic and pulmonic valves thus creates the second heart sound, S2, and diastole begins. The systolic pulmonary pressure is about one-fifth of that of the systemic circulation [5].

7.4 The Cardiovascular Exam

A thorough assessment of a patient's medical status is paramount prior to providing dental care. With regard to the cardiovascular portion of the assessment, it begins with a complete investigation of the patient's *medical history*. Positive responses to any of the following warrant medical consultation or referral:

- Any history of congenital heart disease, syndromes associated with congenital heart defects, or other extracardiac congenital anomalies places the patient at higher risk of cardiovascular issues. Genetic disorders associated with cardiovascular malformations include Down syndrome, Turner syndrome, DiGeorge syndrome, Williams syndrome, VATER/VACTERL association, CHARGE syndrome, Ehlers-Danlos syndrome, Marfan syndrome, and Noonan syndrome [5, 6].
- The history should include pointed questions about any signs or symptoms of cardiac compromise. All patients should be questioned regarding their physical stamina. In infants, lethargy, respiratory symptoms, irritability, and cyanosis are concerning, while nonspecific, signs of cardiac disease. Feeding

intolerance with poor weight gain is also common in infants with significant cardiac disease since feeding is one of the most likely "stressors" to which the infant is exposed [2, 7]. In older children, syncope, chest pain, shortness of breath, poor weight gain, and low energy levels or a low tolerance for exercise are red flags [7]. There are myriad causes of childhood syncope, many of which are benign. However, syncope associated with exercise, chest pain, diagnosed heart disease, or a family history of arrhythmias or sudden cardiac death is worrisome for structural or electrical heart disease [2]. Palpitations are an unpleasant awareness of one's heartbeat [3]. Older children and young adults may be able to report such sensations, often using terms such as "skipping," "fluttering," "flip-flopping," and "racing." Palpitations can indicate an irregular heartbeat, increased strength of contraction, or rapid rate changes; they are not always pathologic but are worth referring for an electrocardiogram [3]. Adopting a squatting posture during play is suggestive of tetralogy of Fallot.

- Past experiences with medical and surgical treatment should be queried, particularly for cardiorespiratory complications or cardiac-related procedures.
- A list of currently prescribed medications and devices can immediately identify cardiovascular disease.
- Family history (parent or sibling) should be determined, particularly for cases of arrhythmia, hypertrophic cardiomyopathy, congenital heart disease, and sudden cardiac death. Hypertrophic cardiomyopathy is inherited in an autosomal dominant pattern but is often asymptomatic [8].

The next step in the assessment of the heart is the *physical exam*. The exam is preferably completed with the patient supine; although with young, active patients, this may be challenging. Components of the physical examination include:

- The general appearance of the patient.
- Baseline vital signs.
- Palpation of arterial pulses.
- Palpation of the precordium.
- Auscultation of the heart sounds.

7.4.1 General Appearance

The general appearance of the patient can be noted by simple observation during the rest of the examination. Features of particular concern include cyanosis, abdominal distension, and clubbing.

Central cyanosis is a blue-purple discoloration of the tissues best identified in the tongue and oral mucosa. It is associated with an oxygen saturation of 85% or less. Cyanosis related to congenital heart disease is most commonly seen in the first weeks of life; patients presenting later with unexplained cyanosis should receive urgent medical attention [2, 9].

Abdominal distension should also be scouted as it is concerning for hepatic or splenic enlargement suggestive of venous congestion. In the case of heart disease, this can occur in the setting of right heart dysfunction when the heart is unable to move the blood forward [2, 4]. Unlike in adult patients, jugular veins and pulsations are difficult to see in children, so they are not used to evaluate volume status and cardiac function [3]. Peripheral edema is an uncommon manifestation of cardiac disease in children; more often it is related to renal disease [2].

Clubbing of the nails can occur in chronic hypoxemia. The tips of the fingers enlarge, the nails start to curve over the fingertips, and the angle at the nail bed is lost. Clubbing is most often bilateral and symmetric. A variety of conditions, including benign ones, can cause clubbing, but in children it is most often associated with congenital heart disease or cystic fibrosis [10].

7.4.2 Baseline Vital Signs and Palpation of Pulses

Vital sign measurements include heart rate, blood pressure, respiratory rate, and temperature and can also include hemoglobin saturation by pulse oximetry [4]. These are particularly important prior to a sedation or general anesthesia visit. If the patient is anxious or agitated, vital signs may be difficult to attain or abnormal. In this setting, checking vital signs in order of least to most uncomfortable, or coming back to vital signs later in the visit, may be helpful.

7.4.2.1 Blood Pressure

An accurate blood pressure measurement depends on selecting the appropriate size cuff for the patient. The width of the cuff should cover two-thirds of the upper arm or leg. The length of the inflatable portion of the cuff should be around 80% of the upper arm circumference [9]. It is preferable that the extremity upon which the cuff is placed is free of clothing. It is important that the artery the cuff is registering be at heart level; if the thigh is being used, the patient should be supine. The blood pressure cuff should fit snugly. Blood pressure readings from the thigh are around 10–20 mmHg higher than those from the upper arm [9, 11, 12]. However, in patients with coarctation of the aorta, blood pressure readings in the upper extremities will be the same or greater than blood pressure readings in the lower extremities. The femoral pulses will also be diminished or delayed [9].

Falsely high readings can occur in the setting of the arm being lower than heart level, the cuff being too loose, and the cuff being too narrow; the opposite can be said for falsely low readings. Blood pressure levels also fluctuate normally over the course of the day, especially in the setting of changes in physical activity, emotional state, pain, and temperature [3]. Causes of sustained hypertension in young children include coarctation of the aorta, renal artery disease and other renal malformations, pheochromocytomas, thyroid disease, and primary hypertension [9, 12]. Causes of hypotension in patients include heart failure, hypovolemia, and shock [12]. Any abnormal blood pressure reading should be confirmed by a subsequent measurement later in the examination. In children, blood pressure categories are based on

Table 7.1 Normal blood pressure values in children [1, 13, 14]

Normal blood pressures (mmHg)			
Age	Systolic pressure	Diastolic pressure	Mean arterial pressure
Neonate	67–84	35–53	45–60
Infant	72–104	37–56	50–62
Toddler	86–104	41–62	50–62
Preschooler	90–112	47–70	58–69
School-aged	94–116	59–78	66–72
Preadolescent	100–120	62–80	71–79
Adolescent	110–129	64–83	73–84

the average blood pressure for age, sex, and height and are reported in percentiles. A child with high blood pressure is in the 95th or higher percentile for that child's age, sex, and height. A child with normal blood pressure is below the 90th percentile [9] (Table 7.1).

7.4.2.2 Heart Rate and Rhythm

Heart rate (Table 7.2) and rhythm can be assessed by pulse oximetry or by palpating pulse points. It is good practice to palpate pulses on a regular basis to gain experience in finding them and confidence in diagnosing an abnormal pulse. Pulses are best felt with the pads of the index and middle fingers. An irregular pulse (one with an abnormal rhythm) should be confirmed by listening to the heart; irregular rhythms are suggestive of dysfunction in the electrical system of the heart. The exception is sinus arrhythmia, in which the rhythm varies regularly and cyclically with respiration. On inspiration, the heart rate accelerates, and with expiration, it decelerates.

An abnormal heart rate and/or irregular heart rhythm can be due to cardiac and noncardiac causes. If suspected, the patient should be referred for medical consultation. The medical referral should be urgent if the patient is experiencing symptoms such as hypotensive episodes, light-headedness, palpitations, and syncope [2, 9]. The concern with cardiac arrhythmias is whether the heart rhythm is stable enough to allow a cardiac output adequate to sustain arterial pressure. Bradycardias may not produce enough cycles to maintain cardiac output, whereas tachycardias may decrease time for ventricular filling and therefore decrease stroke volume [4]. Supraventricular tachycardias are more likely with heart rates $\geq$180 in children and $\geq$220 in infants and are corroborated by a history of abrupt initiation of the tachycardia, invariable heart rate during the tachycardia, and abnormal or absent P waves on ECG [9]. Bradycardia is defined as a heart rate less than 100 beats per minute in children less than 3 years old and less than 60 beats per minutes in children 3–9 years old [9].

Causes of tachycardia in children [2]

- Common causes: fever, crying, anxiety, pain, anemia
- Life-threatening cardiac conditions: supraventricular tachycardia/ventricular tachycardia/other arrhythmias, hypertrophic cardiomyopathy, myocarditis
- Other causes: hyperthyroidism, acute rheumatic fever, Kawasaki disease

Table 7.2 Normal heart rate values in children

Normal heart rates (beats per minute)		
Age	Awake rate	Sleeping rate
Neonate	100–205	90–160
Infant	100–170	75–160
Toddler	90–150	70–120
Preschooler	80–130	65–100
School-aged	70–118	60–90
Adolescent	60–90	50–90

Causes of bradycardia in children [2]

- Cardiac: atrial septal defect and/or its repair, atrioventricular canal, long QT syndrome, Brugada syndrome
- Medications: beta blockers, calcium channel blockers, clonidine, opioids
- Other: systemic lupus erythematosus, hypothermia (<35 °C), vasovagal syncope, sleep

In additional to identifying heart rate and rhythm, pulses can also be used to assess a patient's general state of perfusion. If coarctation of the aorta is suspected in a patient, comparing the timing and intensity of the right brachial and femoral pulses simultaneously can aid in diagnosis. Femoral pulses can be weak in coarctation of the aorta patients [5, 7]. Diffusely diminished pulses are related to decreased cardiac output, seen in conditions such as myocardial dysfunction, cardiac tamponade, and obstructive lesions. Bounding pulses are related to a large difference between systolic and diastolic pressure and are classically seen in aortic regurgitation [5].

7.4.2.3 Pulse Oximetry

Pulse oximetry detects heart rate (noted above) as well as the percent of oxygen saturation of hemoglobin in the blood (oxygen saturation, or SpO_2). An oxygen saturation of 94% or lower in an awake child at sea level is considered abnormal, and the saturation should be confirmed via a second reading. Of note, pulse oximeters may not function well on cold extremities; when the patient is moving; in certain types of light; and on black, blue, or green nail polish [15]. Hypoxemia, as suggested by a low oxygen saturation, can have a pulmonary or cardiac etiology, although many children with heart disease have normal oxygen saturations. A consistently low pulse oximetry reading justifies a medical consultation.

7.4.3 Auscultation of Heart Sounds and Palpation of the Precordium

It is helpful for the examiner to create a routine of listening to all components of the cardiac cycle. For instance, the practitioner can identify the normal heart sounds first, noting the effects of respiration. Next, focus can be turned to murmurs, concentrating on systole and then diastole [16]. The examiner can then return to any areas that sound abnormal and listen to adjacent regions to determine where the sounds are loudest and where they radiate [3]. The shallow bell of the stethoscope is used to hear low frequencies, whereas the diaphragm is used for high frequencies such as S1 and S2. Some stethoscopes incorporate these two functions into one surface so the amount of pressure against the chest determines whether the stethoscope picks up low or high frequencies [17].

1. Palpation of the chest to assess precordial activity.

    Increased precordial activity is commonly felt in patients with increased right or left ventricular stroke volume, such as those with an atrial septal defect or moderate to large ventricular septal defect. The differential for increased precordial activity includes hyperthyroidism, anemia, and anxiety [7]. Precordial palpation is also used to detect thrills, which are palpable vibrations caused by blood flowing rapidly from high to low pressure areas. Thrills feel like the throat of a purring cat [3]. Thrills are typically caused by pathologic lesions, for example, a ventricular septal defect may result in a thrill felt at the lower left sternal border [7].

2. Auscultation of First (S1) and Second (S2) Heart Sounds in All Four Listening Areas

    Thorough cardiac auscultation includes listening in the principal areas of the heart: tricuspid, pulmonary, mitral, and aortic. These areas do overlap (please refer to Fig. 7.3).

   - Tricuspid area (between right atrium and right ventricle): lower left sternal border, specifically the fourth and fifth intercostal spaces along the left sternal edge.
   - Pulmonary area (between the right ventricle and pulmonary artery): second and third intercostal spaces along the left sternal border.

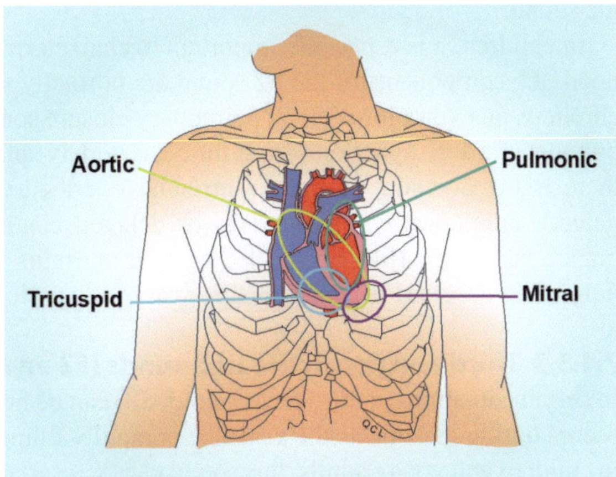

Fig. 7.3 Listening areas of the heart

- Mitral area (between left atrium and left ventricle): fifth intercostal space in the midclavicular line, involves the cardiac apex.
- Aortic area (between the left ventricle and aorta): second intercostal space along the right sternal border and extending to the suprasternal area.

7.4.3.1 First Heart Sound (S1)

The first heart sound (S1) is generated by the closure of the atrioventricular valves (mitral and tricuspid) during early systole, or more specifically, during isovolumetric ventricular contraction [16]. It corresponds to the QRS complex on ECG [5]. The sound is best heard in the mitral and tricuspid areas at the lower left sternal border with extension to the midclavicular line. The interval between the first and second heart sounds is shorter than the interval between the second heart sound and the subsequent first heart sound; for this reason, the identification of which heart sound is which is easier at lower heart rates. At about a rate of 120 beats per minute, the durations of systole and diastole become indistinguishable. In this case, palpation of the carotid pulse or apical impulse is helpful, since those occur in systole right after S1 [16].

7.4.3.2 Second Heart Sound (S2)

The second heart sound (S2) is generated by the closure of the semilunar valves (aortic and pulmonary) during late systole, or more specifically, when the pressure in the ventricles fall following ventricular contraction and ejection of blood. Generally, the S2 is comprised of a louder and earlier aortic valve closing sound (A2) followed closely by the pulmonary valve closing sound (P2). This split in the second heart sound is most obvious (and normal) during inspiration and is termed normal physiologic splitting when auscultated [16]. The mechanism is decreased intrathoracic pressure during inspiration leading to increased blood volume returning to the right heart. When the right ventricle is filled more than the left, it takes slightly longer to empty and causes the pulmonary valve to close later. Effects of inspiration on the left side of the heart are the opposite [5, 16]. The normal split of S2 during inspiration is 0.05 s [5]. During expiration, A2 and P2 fuse into a single sound.

In children, it is especially important to characterize the S2 sound. During childhood, the components of the S2 sound are normally split with inspiration and synchronous on expiration. A loud pulmonary closure sound suggests the possibility of pulmonary artery hypertension. If the S2 is widely split or is split in a fixed manner, there is the potential of right ventricular overload (such as seen in atrial septal defect), pulmonary valve stenosis, or delayed conduction (such as right bundle branch block) [5, 16]. Right-sided cardiac murmurs are accentuated with inspiration, whereas left-sided abnormalities vary little with the respiratory cycle [16].

7.4.3.3 Third and Fourth Heart Sounds (S3 and S4)

In certain situations, a third heart sound, S3, can be heard following S2. This sound occurs during diastole as the ventricle is rapidly filling with blood from the atrium. In children and young adults, this sound can be a variant of normal since their hearts are less compliant. In patients over the age of 40, an "S3 gallop" is generally a sign of enlarged ventricles [3, 5, 17]. S3 is best auscultated with the bell of the stethoscope. The cadence of the sound is "Ken-tuc-ky" with S1 being "Ken," S2 being "tuc," and S3 being "ky" [5, 17].

A fourth heart sound, S4, is also a sign of pathology. It is heard immediately preceding S1 and marks atrial contraction [3]. It is produced as blood enters a stiff ventricle, such as seen in ventricular hypertrophy. S4 is associated with the P wave on ECG and is also best heard with the bell of the stethoscope. The cadence of the sound is "Ten-nes-see" with S4 being "Ten," S1 being "nes," and S2 being "see" [5, 17].

3. Auscultation of Heart Murmurs in all four listening areas

Once S1 and S2 have been identified, focus can be turned to listening for heart murmurs in the same four listening areas. Heart murmurs are a sign of turbulent blood flow, but not all murmurs are indicative of structural or physiological pathology [16]. Murmurs are distinguishable from heart sounds by their longer duration [3]. Murmurs are classified according to the following characteristics.

7.4.4 Classification of Heart Murmurs [16]

(a) Timing—the relationship to S1 and S2, systolic or diastolic
(b) Intensity—loudness
   - Grade 1: barely audible, heard only with intense concentration
   - Grade 2: faint, but heard quickly
   - Grade 3: easily heard, intermediate intensity
   - Grade 4: easily heard, with an associated thrill (a palpable vibration felt on the chest)
   - Grade 5: very loud, with an associated thrill
   - Grade 6: extremely loud, audible with the stethoscope off the chest wall
     *All murmurs louder than grade 3 are pathologic [7].
(c) Location—location on the chest where the sound is loudest and full area over which the sound is audible (radiation).

7.4.4.1 Murmur Areas [5, 7]
The presumable cause of a murmur can be determined by identifying the region where the murmur is loudest.

Upper right sternal border → aortic stenosis, venous hum

Upper left sternal border → pulmonary stenosis, pulmonary flow murmur (benign), atrial septal defect, patent ductus arteriosus

Lower left sternal border → Still's murmur (benign), ventricular septal defect, tricuspid valve regurgitation, hypertrophic cardiomyopathy, subaortic stenosis

Apex → mitral valve regurgitation

The duration, shape, or configuration of the murmur, pitch, and quality of harmonics and overtones can also be categorized during more complete cardiovascular examinations.

7.4.4.2 Systolic Murmurs

Systolic murmurs start with or follow S1 and end before S2. They can be benign or caused by blood flow across an outflow tract (pulmonary or aortic), atrial or ventricular septal defects, atrioventricular valve regurgitation, or patent ductus arteriosus [7]. Holosystolic, or pansystolic, murmurs start immediately with S1 and continue at the same intensity until S2. They indicate valve regurgitation or large ventricular septal defects [5]. Ejection murmurs are crescendo-decrescendo murmurs (start soft, become louder, then become soft again in association with the amount of blood flow during ventricular systole). Innocent murmurs are often ejection systolic. This type of murmur can also represent narrowing of the aortic or pulmonary valves/outflow tracts (e.g., aortic stenosis) [5]. Early systolic murmurs start immediately with S1 but taper and stop before S2. These represent small muscular ventricular septal defects [5]. Mid to late systolic murmurs begin at the midpoint of systole and can represent regurgitation from mitral valve prolapse, especially when heard in association with a preceding mid-systolic click [7].

7.4.4.3 Diastolic Murmurs

Diastole is the period between the closure of the aortic and pulmonary valves and the closure of the tricuspid and mitral valves. Diastolic murmurs fall between S2 and S1 and generally represent pathology [3]. Diastole is usually quiet because the low-pressure flow through relatively large valves creates little turbulence. Turbulence can occur, however, with valvular heart disease such as semilunar valve regurgitation or atrioventricular valve stenosis [3, 5, 16].

7.4.4.4 Continuous Murmurs

Flow through vessels or channels beyond the aortic and pulmonary valves is not confined by systole and diastole, and turbulent flow can therefore be heard throughout the cardiac cycle. Such murmurs usually are pathologic (e.g., patent ductus arteriosus), but the venous hum is a notable exception (refer to section 7.4.4.8) [5, 16].

7.4.4.5 Pericardial Friction Rub

Pericarditis is inflammation or infection of the membrane surrounding the heart. A pericardial friction rub occurs when inflamed pericardial surfaces rub against each other during the movement of the heart within its pericardial sac [17]. This creates a scratching or grating sound, like rubbing two pieces of sandpaper together, that can be present in both systole and diastole. The sound is heard best at the left sternal border during inspiration. The most common causes of pericarditis in children are viral infection and sequelae from heart surgery [6]. Associated symptoms include chest pain, fever, irritability, fatigue, and irregular heart rhythm.

7.4.4.6 Still's Murmur

The most common innocent murmur in childhood is the vibratory murmur described by physician George Still in 1909 [16]. It is found most typically between the ages of 2 and 6 years but can present earlier and last later into adolescence. The pitch is described as low to medium, and the sound is characterized as musical with multiple overtones. As Dr. Still explained, it resembles "a twanging sound, very like that made by twanging a piece of tense string" [9, 16]. It has also been characterized as sounding like a "jar of bumblebees with their wings fluttering" [5]. The intensity of the murmur is grade 3 or less; therefore, there is no palpable thrill. The intensity of the murmur diminishes, and the character changes, with upright positioning. It is maximal along the mid to lower left sternal boarder and extends to the cardiac apex. This murmur can be extremely variable and is accentuated in states of increased cardiac output, such as fever or anxiety [9]. The origin of the murmur is not entirely clear. It has been attributed to the vibration of pulmonary valves during systolic ejection, to the movement of blood in a contracting ventricle, to narrowing of the left ventricular outflow tract, and to the presence of false tendons in the ventricles [16].

While a Still's murmur will decrease in intensity when the patient stands, most pathologic murmurs will not change significantly. The murmur of hypertrophic cardiomyopathy is an exception, as it *increases* in intensity when the patient stands. This phenomenon occurs because of decreased venous return to the heart when standing. This leads to decreased left ventricular volume, which in turn, increases the left ventricular outflow tract narrowing and obstruction, and hence the murmur. Hypertrophic cardiomyopathy is rare, but it is one of the leading causes of sudden death in young athletes [7].

7.4.4.7 Pulmonary Flow Murmur

A benign murmur of the pulmonary outflow tract can be heard in children up until young adulthood [16]. The sound is described as rough and dissonant and is of a grade 2 or 3 intensity. It occurs in early-to mid-systole. The murmur is heard at the upper left sternal border (pulmonary area). Like Still's murmur, it is best heard in the supine position and should not be associated with a palpable thrill. It is augmented by full exhalation.

To distinguish this benign murmur from pathology [16]:

- The murmur of an atrial septal defect occurs because of increased blood flow through the pulmonary outflow tract and can sound very similar. With this defect, there may be an accompanying hyperdynamic right ventricular impulse, wide fixed splitting of the S2, and a mid-diastolic flow rumble.
- The murmur of pulmonary valve stenosis can be differentiated from that of a benign pulmonary flow murmur by the presence of a systolic thrill, its higher pitch and longer duration, and a widely split S2. Pulmonary valve stenosis can also cause an ejection click due to improper opening of the stenotic valve.

7.4.4.8 Venous Hum

This innocent murmur is the most common continuous murmur heard in children. It is best heard at the lower anterior portion of the neck just lateral to the sternocleidomastoid muscle and inferiorly in the area just below the right clavicle. The sound is loudest on the right, when the patient is sitting rather than supine, and in diastole. It is described as hollow, whining, roaring, or whirring, and patients may be aware of it. The intensity varies from quite faint to very loud. The venous hum is best elicited with the patient sitting with head turned away from the examiner. Turning the head toward the side of the murmur or applying light pressure on the jugular vein (decreasing venous return) can decrease or eliminate the sound [9]. These benign murmurs can have the same quality as breath sounds, which makes them more difficult to recognize [9]. Venous hums are caused by the flow of venous blood from the head and neck to the thorax, when there is turbulence either at the confluence of the internal jugular and subclavian veins with the superior vena cava or in the internal jugular vein as it travels across the transverse process of the atlas [16]. While venous hums are normal, all other diastolic murmurs are pathologic and warrant referral [7].

7.4.5   Atrial Septal Defects

Because of the prevalence of atrial septal defects (ASDs) in the population, and because it is a frequently missed diagnosis [7], it is worth spending extra time learning the clinical findings of this particular anomaly. Indeed, symptoms associated with ASDs are uncommon or subtle in children, and some ASDs are not diagnosed until adulthood [6]. The abnormalities detected in patients with ASDs are similar to those found in patients with innocent murmurs, but the two can be differentiated. Murmurs from ventricular septal defects (VSDs) or significant valvular stenosis are not so subtle and less likely to be attributed to an innocent murmur [7]. The following are factors that help differentiate innocent murmurs from those associated with an ASD [7]:

- Precordial activity. Right ventricular enlargement can occur in the setting of an ASD, which leads to increased precordial activity felt by palpation at the left sternal border.
- Auscultation of S2 splitting. When listening at the upper left sternal border, a widely split S2 that doesn't change with the respiratory cycle is indicative of an ASD. An ASD leads to an increased volume of blood in the right ventricle, and the right ventricle will therefore take longer to empty with the pulmonary valve closing later. In young children, it can be challenging to determine the respiratory variation of S2 splitting. By preschool age, the abnormal splitting of S2 generally becomes clear [7], although the cooperation and activity level of the patient may still make auscultation difficult.
- Location where the murmur is best heard. The systolic murmur of an ASD is caused by the increased blood volume traveling across the right ventricular outflow tract (pulmonary valve) from right ventricular volume overload due to

left-to-right shunting; it is best heard at the upper left sternal border [6]. Generally, an innocent Still's murmur is heard best at the lower left sternal border. An innocent pulmonary flow murmur may be heard in the same location as the ASD murmur, however.

- Presence of a diastolic murmur. ASDs can cause a quiet rumbling sound in diastole because of increased diastolic blood flow across the tricuspid valve; this sound is best heard with the bell of the stethoscope held gently on the lower left sternal border. A venous hum is an innocent murmur that is heard in diastole, but it is distinct in its location and diminishment with patient head movement toward the side of the exam.
- Change in the murmur when the patient stands. In a patient with an ASD, the increased precordial activity, widely split S2, upper left sternal border systolic murmur, and diastolic rumble at the lower left sternal border should all remain. In a patient with an innocent murmur, the systolic murmur should diminish in intensity upon standing [7].

Summary of Differences Between an Atrial Septal Defect Murmur and an Innocent Murmur [7]

Precordial activity → normal in an innocent murmur, increased in ASD

S1 → normal in both

S2 → physiological splitting with respiratory cycle in an innocent murmur, widely split and fixed in ASD

Systolic murmur (supine) → likely crescendo/decrescendo in both but vibratory at lower left sternal border in innocent and flow at upper left sternal border in ASD

Systolic murmur (standing) → decreases in intensity in innocent, doesn't change in ASD

Diastolic murmur → venous hum in innocent, rumble across tricuspid valve in ASD

7.5 Integrating Examination Findings

7.5.1 Murmur Evaluation in the Pediatric Patient

When evaluating a patient for a murmur, it is important to remember that, outside of the newborn period, a normal murmur can be detected in the majority of children [6]. These murmurs can be detected at any age—although usually between 1 and 14 years—and are often intermittent [18]. Furthermore, the incidence of serious congenital heart disease is below 1%, and most of said disease is identified before 3 months of age [5, 8]. Structural heart disease is found in approximately 10% of children having a murmur, with ventricular septal defect being the most common lesion [6]. Pulmonary valve stenosis and atrial septal defects are the next most common lesions [6]. Murmurs detected for the first time after 1 year of age most often are innocent murmurs but can represent valve stenosis or regurgitation, or atrial septal defects. A new murmur in a patient with a history of recent streptococcal pharyngitis could represent rheumatic fever with cardiac involvement, which usually effects the left-heart valves (mitral > aortic) [5].

While correctly identifying congenital heart disease requires a broad knowledge of cardiac anatomy and physiology and the nuances of heart sounds, in most children with cardiac disease, there will be a constellation of findings that represent the disease process (Table 7.3) [2]. Therefore, to help differentiate an innocent murmur from pathology, we return to the previously completed medical history, which will aid in identifying children at increased risk for significant heart disease. The following findings warrant referral for further cardiac assessment [16]:

- Children with chromosomal disorders known to have a higher incidence of structural cardiac abnormalities (Down syndrome, Turner syndrome, DiGeorge syndrome, CHARGE, VATER, etc.)
- The existence of congenital abnormalities in other organ systems, which are associated with structural anomalies in the heart in up to a quarter of patients.
- Perinatal history of prematurity, maternal diabetes, toxin ingestion, or fetal distress.
- A family history (parent or sibling) of hypertrophic cardiomyopathy, congenital heart disease, or unexplained sudden death of a family member.
- Patients who report cardiac symptoms such as decreased capacity for exercise or play, syncope, chest pain, palpitations, or shortness of breath.

Table 7.3 Factors that distinguish cardiac pathology from a benign condition [5, 7, 8]

	Factors associated with cardiac disease	Factors associated with a benign condition
Medical history	Parent or sibling with congenital heart disease (CHD) or sudden death	Negative family history
	Prenatal maternal condition associated with CHD (e.g., diabetes, PKU, multifetal pregnancy)	Non-syndromic
	Underlying genetic disorder associated with CHD (e.g., down syndrome, DiGeorge syndrome)	Age >2 years
	Age <1 year	Asymptomatic
	Symptoms: respiratory difficulties, syncope, cyanosis, chest pain, etc.	
Murmur	Grade intensity of ≥3	Grade <3 intensity
	Holosystolic timing	Short systolic timing
	Harsh or blowing	Musical or vibratory
	Increased intensity with upright position (or no change)	Softer intensity with patient sitting compared to supine
	Diastolic	Minimal radiation
	Abnormal S2	Normal S2
	Gallop rhythm (S3 or S4)	No gallop, click, or rub
	Systolic click	
Other physical exam findings	Abnormal vital signs (e.g. bradycardia, tachycardia, BP gradient)	Normal vital signs
	Abnormal pulses (e.g. diminished pulses especially femoral, bounding pulses)	Normal pulses
	Hepatomegaly	No other findings
	Extracardiac congenital anomalies	

A clinician's assessment of the heart will likely take on extra significance when considering a patient for sedation or anesthesia. The primary risk factors for mortality during surgery are cyanosis, younger age, more complex cardiac defects, poor general health, and current treatment for cardiac failure [8]. Patients who have undergone corrective surgery for less complex lesions (e.g., atrial septal defect, ventricular septal defect, patent ductus arteriosus) and are well-compensated do not have an increased risk for mortality during subsequent surgery [8]. However, consultation with the patient's cardiologist is strongly recommended in such cases prior to considering sedation.

Upon referral, additional studies that help elucidate cardiac abnormalities may be ordered, including chest radiography, echocardiogram, and electrocardiogram. Chest radiography is a well-tolerated test that can help differentiate cardiac from pulmonary pathology and help diagnose certain heart defects. Echocardiography is the standard for establishing the cause of a murmur. In current clinical practice, it is indicated in patients with cardiac symptoms plus a murmur and in any patient with a diastolic murmur, grade intensity murmur of >3, or a murmur in association with any other abnormal findings on examination [19]. Electrocardiograms help diagnose irregularities in heart rate and rhythm and also enlargement of the heart chambers [8]. In an ideal world, in the event a new murmur is detected in an asymptomatic, otherwise healthy child, diagnostic studies are unlikely to alter the diagnosis of a benign murmur when made by an experienced clinician. However, without thorough training and practice in auscultation, and in the setting of uncooperative or active pediatric patients, it is often difficult to make a confident diagnosis. Referral to a pediatrician or pediatric cardiologist is indicated and valid in this setting.

References

1. Milnes AR, Wilson S. Preoperative assessment and review of systems. In: Wilson S, editor. Oral sedation for dental procedures in children. Springer; 2015. p. 25–37.
2. Kane DA. Suspected heart disease in infants and children: criteria for referral. In: Fulton DR, Lorin MI, Armsby C, editors. UpToDate. UpToDate; 2021.
3. Szilagyi PG. The cardiovascular system. In: Bickley L, editor. Bates' guide to physical examination and history taking. 9th ed. Lippincott Williams & Wilkins; 2007. p. 279–335.
4. Becker DE. Preoperative medical evaluation: part 1: general principles and cardiovascular considerations. Anesth Prog. 2009;56:92–103.
5. Geggel RL. Approach to the infant or child with a cardiac murmur. In: Fulton DR, Lorin MI, Armsby C, editors. UpToDate. UpToDate; 2021.
6. Geggel RL. Common causes of cardiac murmurs in infants and children. In: Fulton DR, Armsby C, editors. UpToDate. UpToDate; 2021.
7. McConnell ME, Adkins SB III, Hannon DW. Heart murmurs in pediatric patients: when do you refer? Am Fam Physician. 1999;60(2):558–64.
8. Bhatia N, Barber N. Dilemmas in preoperative assessment of children. Contin Educ Anesth Crit Care Pain. 2011;11(6):214–8.
9. Szilagyi PG. Assessing children: infancy through adolescence. In: Bickley L, editor. Bates' guide to physical examination and history taking. 9th ed. Lippincott Williams & Wilkins; 2007. p. 279–335.

10. Huffman GB. Clubbing: bedside evaluation for associated conditions. Am Fam Physician. 2002;65(9):1907–11.
11. Szilagyi PG. Beginning the physical examination: general survey and vital signs. In: Bickley L, editor. Bates' guide to physical examination and history taking. 9th ed. Lippincott Williams & Wilkins; 2007. p. 89–120.
12. Drutz JE. The pediatric physical examination: general principles and standard measurements. In: Duryea TK, Torchia MM, editors. UpToDate. UpToDate; 2020.
13. American Heart Association and American Association of Critical Care Nurses. PALS digital reference card. 2016.
14. University of Iowa Carver College of Medicine Department of Otolaryngology. Pediatric vital signs normal ranges. 2023. https://medicine.uiowa.edu/iowaprotocols/pediatric-vital-signs-normal-ranges. Accessed 30 Mar 2023.
15. Cote CJ, Goldstein EA, Fuchsman WH, Hoaglin DC. The effect of nail polish on pulse oximetry. Anesth Analg. 1988;6(7):683–6.
16. Pelech AN. The cardiac murmur: when to refer? Pediatr Clin N Am. 1998;45(1):107–22. https://doi.org/10.1016/s0031-3955(05)70585-x.
17. Meyer TE. Auscultation of heart sounds. In: Gersh BJ, Yeon SB, editors. UpToDate. UpToDate; 2021.
18. Cardiac Murmur (R01.1). Pediatric cardiology management and referral guidelines, Dell Children's Medical Center of Central Texas.
19. Gersh BJ. Physiologic and pharmacologic maneuvers in the differential diagnosis of heart murmurs. In: Otto CM, Yeon SB, editors. UpToDate. UpToDate; 2021.

Assessment of the Gut

8

Sherief Mansi and Ajay Kaul

8.1 Introduction

The gastrointestinal tract (GIT) is one of the largest organs in the body. The oral-gut health connection cannot be emphasized enough. GIT disease can have manifestations in the oral cavity like in inflammatory bowel disease (IBD) and celiac disease [1, 2] similar to many systemic diseases that may involve multiple organs or body parts. It is important for dentists to be aware of this oral-gut connection to be able to identify conditions that may directly or indirectly impact the treatment plan. The oral cavity may act as a mirror reflecting what is happening distally in the gut. Dentists must be aware of the most common gastrointestinal disease manifestations in the oral cavity.

The index of suspicion is very important in identifying disease pathology to be able to do the appropriate workup and referral for any medical specialist. The oral cavity is the main focus of attention during a dental visit, and a comprehensive approach to the patient's health may be unintentionally missed. Diagnosis starts with good history taking and a thorough physical exam which may be overlooked in the patient's dental visit. Indeed, the identification of risk factors and red flags during history taking and physical examination is essential for diagnosing certain gastrointestinal diseases as well as avoiding potential complications during dental procedures. This chapter will focus on the important aspects of the patient's medical history and physical examination to achieve this goal.

S. Mansi · A. Kaul (✉)
Division of Gastroenterology, Cincinnati Children's Hospital/University of Cincinnati, Cincinnati, OH, USA
e-mail: Sherief.mansi@cchmc.org; Ajay.kaul@cchmc.org

8.2 Medical History

One of the most important aspects of any clinical encounter is a thorough history taking by the provider regardless of his or her specialty as the body acts as one integrated unit. There are many different clues and red flags that the dentist can identify with good history taking with regard to GIT pathology. Below we will discuss in details important questions that should be asked during a pediatric patient encounter and how they may help in the patient's management.

8.2.1 Family History and Past Medical History

General questions regarding the patient's family history and past medical history should target the identification of generalized physical illnesses as well as specific GIT pathology. We will give a background on some GIT that are relevant to a pediatric dentist.

8.2.2 History of Autoimmune Conditions

IBD including both Crohn's disease (CD) and ulcerative colitis (UC) affects different parts of the gut and presents usually with chronic diarrhea, hematochezia (rectal bleeding), weight loss, and abdominal pain [3]. It is commonly associated with oral lesions which are more common in males and children. They are also more common with Crohn's disease than ulcerative colitis [4]. Recurrent oral aphthous ulcers can be seen years before IBD onset and may be related to gut flare-ups. The lesions may have a fluctuating course with some improving quickly and some persisting for a longer period of time. In addition, granulomatous invasion of the oral cavity can occur with CD. Folate and iron deficiency as well as vitamin B12 deficiencies can be seen in patients with IBD possibly due to malabsorption. Folate deficiency is commonly seen with sulfasalazine or methotrexate treatment [5]. Medications used in IBD can cause side effects that may manifest in the oral cavity. Oral lichen planus has been reported with 5-ASA [4]. Gingival hyperplasia has been reported with cyclosporine. Tacrolimus does not usually cause lesions in the oral cavity. Biological agents like anti TNFs can be associated with opportunistic infections like oral candidiasis and HSV ulcers [4].

Celiac disease (also known as celiac sprue) is an autoimmune condition which causes small intestine villi damage due to an immune response to gluten. Close to half of the patients with celiac disease do not present with digestive symptoms at the time of diagnosis (like abdominal pain, bloating, and chronic diarrhea) [3]. Extra-intestinal manifestations include oral manifestations, short stature, iron deficiency anemia, and abnormal liver functions [6]. Celiac disease is more common in patients with other autoimmune disorders like diabetes mellitus type 1 and autoimmune thyroid disease. In addition, it is more common in patients with certain genetic conditions like Down syndrome and Turner syndrome [7]. Serological screening in those high-risk groups is indicated, and a referral to a gastroenterologist may be warranted if there are concerns. Treatment is with a life-long gluten-free diet [7, 8]. Recurrent aphthous stomatitis, atrophic glossitis, glossodynia (tongue pain), oral lichen planus, enamel hypoplasia, dental caries, and delayed tooth eruption have also been described with celiac disease [3, 8, 9].

8.2.3 History of Malabsorption

If there is a history of chronic diarrhea or malnutrition, this may be a clue for vitamin deficiencies. Chronic diarrheal conditions like IBD, celiac disease, and chronic gastrointestinal infections may cause nutrient deficiencies that can manifest in the oral cavity.

Fat-soluble vitamin (A, D, E, K) malabsorption can be seen in severe liver disease (especially with obstructive jaundice) [10] where fat absorption is impaired. Vitamin A deficiency presents with xerostomia. Vitamin D, which is involved in calcium homeostasis, plays an important role in teeth development. Vitamin D deficiency can cause enamel hypoplasia and dentin defects as well as maxillary bone maldevelopment [11]. These changes are usually seen with severe deficiencies involving bones elsewhere in the body [10]. Vitamin E deficiency usually does not have oral manifestations but manifest commonly with neurological symptoms. Vitamin K deficiency typically does not have specific oral manifestations, but prolonged bleeding can be seen during a dental procedure due to prolongation of the prothrombin time (PT) as many coagulation factors produced by the liver are vitamin K dependent [10].

Water-soluble vitamin deficiency can present in the oral cavity as well. Generally, vitamin B complex deficiencies manifest generally in the oral cavity with glossitis, angular stomatitis, painful vesicular eruption and ulceration (seen with thiamine "B1" deficiency), and oculo-orogenital syndrome (conjunctivitis, photophobia, and perineal pruritus seen with riboflavin or vitamin B2 deficiency). Vitamin C deficiency presents with scurvy (gingival edema, bleeding, and loose teeth) [10].

Certain mineral deficiencies can also present in the oral cavity. Iron deficiency usually presents with similar symptoms as vitamin B complex deficiency (glossitis and stomatitis). Severe calcium deficiency has similar oral cavity manifestations as severe vitamin D deficiency. Zinc deficiency can manifest with glossitis, angular stomatitis, perioral dermatitis (usually spares the upper lip), xerostomia, and hypogeusia (loss of taste sensation). Acrodermatitis enteropathica (which is an autosomal recessive disorder) affects zinc absorption and presents with periorificial dermatitis, alopecia, and diarrhea [12]. All mineral deficiencies can be seen with decreased intake (feeding disorder) or malabsorption and chronic diarrheal illnesses.

8.2.4 History of Gastroesophageal Reflux Disease (GERD), Chest Pain and Eating Disorders

Recurrent regurgitation of gastric contents into the mouth can potentially cause dental erosions [13–15]. This is due to the effect of the stomach acid on the enamel with prevalence of dental erosion reaching 70–90% in patients with GERD with primary and permanent dentition respectively depending on the severity of reflux [16]. GERD may present classically with recurrent upper abdomen and/or chest pain (which may be related to eating), heartburn, and belching. Patients with esophageal motility disorders like achalasia or weak peristalsis can have severe GERD that may affect the teeth [3]. However, silent GERD may be hard to identify as it is asymptomatic and it may only present with posterior dental erosions [13]. Mucositis, aphthous-like lesions, and burning sensation in the oral cavity have also been reported [3]. Halitosis (or bad breath) has been reported in patients with GERD and eating disorders [17–19] with active regurgitation of gastric contents in addition to bad oral hygiene. However, no association was found between halitosis and functional dyspepsia or *Helicobacter pylori* infections alone without GERD [20].

8.2.5 History of Liver Disease and GI Bleeding

Green discoloration of the teeth has been reported in patients with severe cholestasis prior to liver transplantation [21]. Apart from oral signs seen with chronic liver disease, there is usually a concern by dentists as well as other surgeons about bleeding in those patients while performing therapeutic or diagnostic procedures. Patients with advanced liver disease and liver failure usually have a balanced deficiency between procoagulant and anticoagulant factors which are affected directly by liver disease [22, 23]. Many studies have reported a poor relationship between laboratory tests like PT/INR and platelets) and the risk for bleeding. In general, it is safe to perform dental procedures including extraction as well as incision and drainage in these patients [22]. Prophylactic transfusion (of platelets and/or fresh frozen plasma) is not indicated before procedures anymore and only indicated for active bleeding. Even platelet counts as low as 16,000 per microliter were safe for dental procedures as long there was no history of active bleeding [24].

Patients with advanced liver disease who have cirrhosis and portal hypertension may have a positive history of upper or lower GI bleeding, but the evaluation of the risk of bleeding is multifactorial and cannot be determined just with lab testing [23]. Patients with solid organ transplant may be on anticoagulation which may influence the decision to perform certain dental procedures.

In general, if an invasive procedure is planned and bleeding is expected, thromboelastography (TEG) is a technique that assesses clot development, stabilization, and dissolution and is used to determine the bleeding status of the patient regardless of the INR level. Major bleeding events are actually rare in patients with chronic liver disease and elevated INR [23, 25]. TEG helps guide product transfusion to prevent excessive bleeding during procedures [25]. Despite this, the guidelines in anesthesiology and interventional radiology literature for bleeding risk in chronic liver disease still rely on INR/PT values. Platelet count and function may have more influence on the risk of bleeding [26]. Consultation of a pediatric hepatologist may be warranted at that time to determine the need for product transfusion before invasive procedures [26, 27].

Other factors to consider in patients with chronic liver disease are medications. Diuretics, which are used commonly in chronic liver disease patients to treat fluid overload, can decrease salivary flow as well as alter its composition, thereby affecting oral health [28].

Isolated lower gastrointestinal bleeding etiology is very diverse and differs slightly with age. This includes polyps, anal fissures (seen commonly with chronic constipation), Meckel's diverticulum in younger patients (usually presents with tarry black stools or melena associated with severe anemia) to infectious, inflammatory disorders (like IBD) in the older population [29]. Most of these disorders are not associated with coagulopathy.

8.2.6 History of Immunosuppression

History of steroid use or other immunosuppressants is important especially in patients with poor oral hygiene. Autoimmune conditions like IBD or autoimmune hepatitis as well as patients with solid organ or intestinal transplant may be associated with chronic steroid use which affects the body immunity. Prompt treatment of dental infections is very important to avoid systemic and potentially fatal complications like sepsis. Opportunistic infections such as oral candidiasis or HSV ulcers (irregular) can be seen with severe immunosuppression. Methotrexate can cause mucositis and ulcerative stomatitis [4]. Cyclosporine has been associated with gingival hyperplasia. Other lesions like enamel hypoplasia and opacity have been reported in posttransplant patients on immunosuppressive agents [21].

8.3 Physical Examination

A thorough physical examination complements good medical history taking in confirming suspected gastrointestinal pathology. It also helps identify red flags that may be missed or were unknown to the patient during history taking.

8.4 Gastrointestinal Tract Conditions that Manifest in the Oral Cavity

1. Glossitis, cheilitis and gingivitis: This can be seen with many vitamin deficiencies such as vitamin B complexes as well as vitamin C, folate deficiency, and severe iron deficiency anemia [10]. For instance, atrophic glossitis presents with

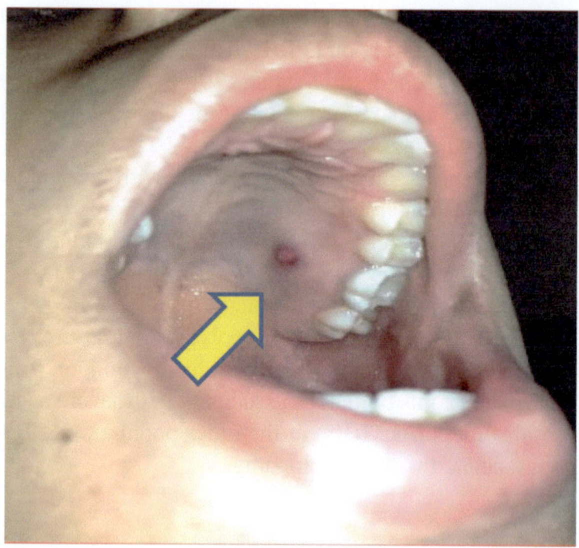

Fig. 8.1 Aphthous ulcer in a patient with Crohn's disease despite having clinical gastrointestinal remission. (Photo courtesy of Dr. Khalil El-Chammas, Cincinnati Children's Hospital Medical Center 'CCHMC', Division of Gastroenterology and Hepatology, Cincinnati, Ohio, USA)

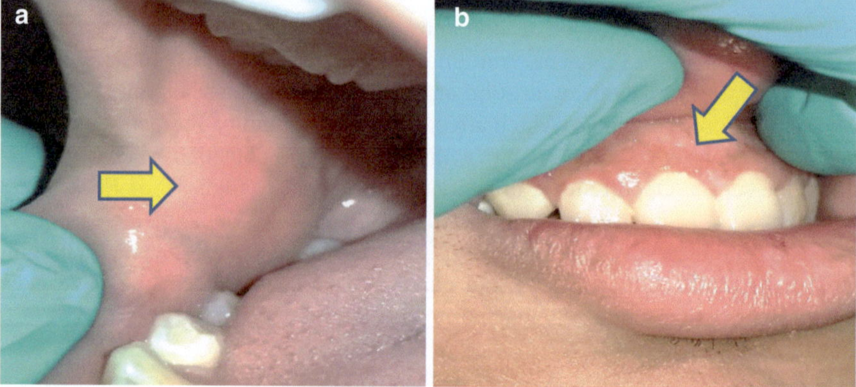

Fig. 8.2 The same patient with clinical gastrointestinal remission of Crohn's disease presenting with oral granulomatous lesions on the buccal surface (**a**) and gingiva (**b**). (Photo courtesy of Dr. Khalil El-Chammas, CCHMC, Division of Gastroenterology and Hepatology, Cincinnati, Ohio, USA)

a glazed, shiny, featureless tongue that may be painful and erythematous. Those lesions can also be seen with IBD [4].

2. Mucosal ulceration: This can be found in autoimmune conditions like inflammatory bowel disease especially Crohn's disease. General involvement of the buccal mucosa has been reported with erythema, ulceration, and sometimes nodularity (Fig. 8.1).

3. Oral granulomas and mucosal ulceration and tags can be seen with Crohn's disease. Cobblestone appearance or raised smooth nodules can be seen that are associated with granulomatous invasion of the buccal mucosa [3, 5]. These

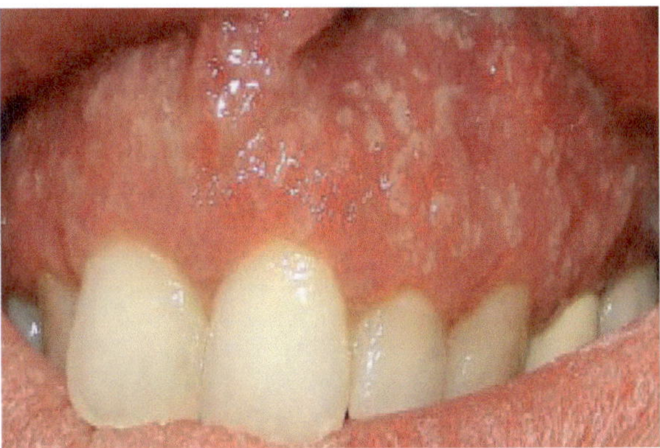

Fig. 8.3 Multiple exophytic pustules on the erythematous base that covered the gingiva and oral mucosa resembling "snail tracks." Microscopic section revealed an intraepithelial clefting and inflammatory cell accumulation (eosinophilic micro-abscesses). The oral lesions recurred as a result of drug discontinuation. [Photo courtesy of *Saede Atarbashi-Moghadam* et al. *Journal of Clinical and Diagnostic Research (2016)*. Reprinted with permission from the publisher, The Journal of Clinical and Diagnostic Research]

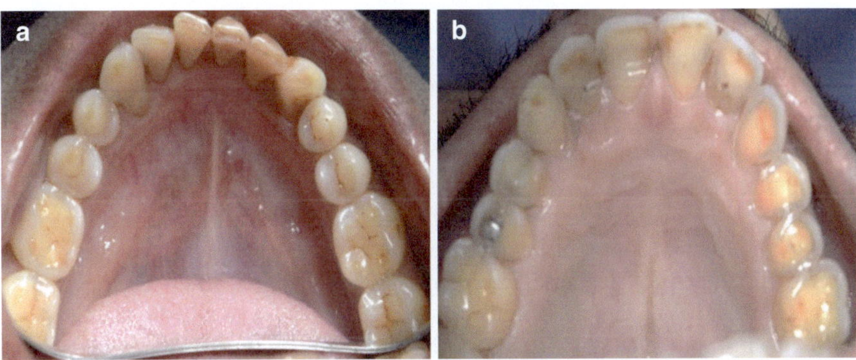

Fig. 8.4 The status of the dentition reveals erosion of the palatal surfaces of the maxillary teeth (**a**) and the occlusal surfaces of the mandibular teeth (**b**). [Photo courtesy of *Sherin Jose Chockattu* et al. *Restor Dent Endod. (2018)*. Reprinted with permission from the author and with unrestricted permission from publisher to reproduce media from current publication as cited properly]

noncaseating granulomas are only seen with Crohn's disease [4]. Swelling of lips and cheeks have also been reported. In severe cases, this can cause deformity [4]. Oral lichen planus has been described with IBD as well as with medications like 5-ASA (even with no sulfa-containing medications like mesalazine) [4] (Fig. 8.2).

4. Pyostomatitis vegetans are multiple eosinophilic pustules (intra- and subepithelial abscesses) seen in the oral cavity that sometimes can form a confluence of lesions resembling a "snail track" [4]. This can be seen in IBD and has been

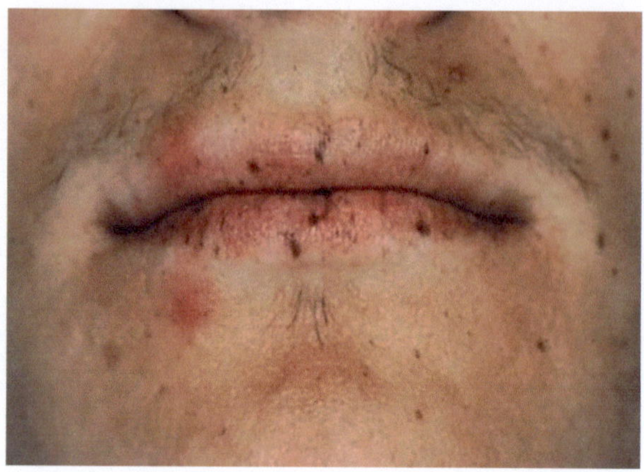

Fig. 8.5 Multiple small, dark brown macules on the lip vermillion and perioral skin of a patient with Peutz-Jeghers syndrome. [Photo courtesy of *Molly S. Rosebush* et al. *Head and Neck Pathology (2019).* Reprinted with permission from Springer nature publications]

described more with UC, and microscopically no granulomas can be seen. It may be considered as the oral equivalent of pyoderma gangrenosum [3] (Fig. 8.3).

5. Dental changes: Those can be seen in conditions like severe vitamin C, D, and calcium deficiencies as well as enamel hypoplasia, dentin defects, and loose teeth [3]. Frequency regurgitation of gastric contents whether due to bulimia or severe gastroesophageal reflux disease (GERD) can manifest with poor dental hygiene and dental erosions. Enamel abnormalities can be seen in celiac disease as well ranging from mild changes to complete disruption of the shape of the tooth (Fig. 8.4).
6. Stomatitis: Candidal stomatitis with white plaques can be seen with immune suppression, e.g., in IBD and posttransplantation of solid organs.
7. Disorders of oral pigmentation: Multiple dark pigmentations seen on the lips may be a manifestation of Peutz-Jeghers syndrome (PJS) which can be associated with other GIT lesions like polyps (Fig. 8.5).

In conclusion, the dental visit should be considered as a complete medical visit despite the focus on the oral cavity which may give clues to disease pathology occurring elsewhere in the gut. This may influence the disease course, treatment, and decision to perform procedures in certain patient. The medical history and physical exam remain the most important tools to achieve a comprehensive diagnostic and therapeutic approach to our patients.

References

1. Crippa R, Zuccotti GV, Mantegazza C. Oral manifestations of gastrointestinal diseases in children. Part 2: Crohn's disease. Eur J Paediatr Dent. 2016;17(2):164–6.
2. Mantegazza C, Paglia M, Angiero F, Crippa R. Oral manifestations of gastrointestinal diseases in children. Part 4: coeliac disease. Eur J Paediatr Dent. 2016;17(4):332–4.
3. Jajam M, Bozzolo P, Niklander S. Oral manifestations of gastrointestinal disorders. J Clin Exp Dent. 2017;9(10):e1242–e8.

4. Muhvic-Urek M, Tomac-Stojmenovic M, Mijandrusic-Sincic B. Oral pathology in inflammatory bowel disease. World J Gastroenterol. 2016;22(25):5655–67.
5. Beitman RG, Frost SS, Roth JL. Oral manifestations of gastrointestinal disease. Dig Dis Sci. 1981;26(8):741.
6. Pastore L, Carroccio A, Compilato D, Panzarella V, Serpico R, Lo Muzio L. Oral manifestations of celiac disease. J Clin Gastroenterol. 2008;42(3):224–32.
7. Hill ID, Dirks MH, Liptak GS, Colletti RB, Fasano A, Guandalini S, et al. Guideline for the diagnosis and treatment of celiac disease in children: recommendations of the North American Society for Pediatric Gastroenterology, Hepatology and Nutrition. J Pediatr Gastroenterol Nutr. 2005;40(1):1–19.
8. Rashid M, Zarkadas M, Anca A, Limeback H. Oral manifestations of celiac disease: a clinical guide for dentists. J Mich Dent Assoc. 2011;93(10):42–6.
9. Ferraz EG, Campos Ede J, Sarmento VA, Silva LR. The oral manifestations of celiac disease: information for the pediatric dentist. Pediatr Dent. 2012;34(7):485–8.
10. Tolkachjov SN, Bruce AJ. Oral manifestations of nutritional disorders. Clin Dermatol. 2017;35(5):441–52.
11. Zambrano M, Nikitakis NG, Sanchez-Quevedo MC, Sauk JJ, Sedano H, Rivera H. Oral and dental manifestations of vitamin D-dependent rickets type I: report of a pediatric case. Oral Surg Oral Med Oral Pathol Oral Radiol Endod. 2003;95(6):705–9.
12. Nistor N, Ciontu L, Frasinariu OE, Lupu VV, Ignat A, Streanga V. Acrodermatitis enteropathica: a case report. Medicine (Baltimore). 2016;95(20):e3553.
13. Ali DA, Brown RS, Rodriguez LO, Moody EL, Nasr MF. Dental erosion caused by silent gastroesophageal reflux disease. J Am Dent Assoc. 2002;133(6):734–7. quiz 68–9.
14. Dahshan A, Patel H, Delaney J, Wuerth A, Thomas R, Tolia V. Gastroesophageal reflux disease and dental erosion in children. J Pediatr. 2002;140(4):474–8.
15. De Oliveira PA, Paiva SM, De Abreu MH, Auad SM. Dental erosion in children with gastroesophageal reflux disease. Pediatr Dent. 2016;38(3):246–50.
16. Taji S, Seow WK. A literature review of dental erosion in children. Aust Dent J. 2010;55(4):358–67. quiz 475.
17. Gaddey HL. Oral manifestations of systemic disease. Gen Dent. 2017;65(6):23–9.
18. Struch F, Schwahn C, Wallaschofski H, Grabe HJ, Volzke H, Lerch MM, et al. Self-reported halitosis and gastro-esophageal reflux disease in the general population. J Gen Intern Med. 2008;23(3):260–6.
19. Lo Russo L, Campisi G, Di Fede O, Di Liberto C, Panzarella V, Lo Muzio L. Oral manifestations of eating disorders: a critical review. Oral Dis. 2008;14(6):479–84.
20. Moshkowitz M, Horowitz N, Leshno M, Halpern Z. Halitosis and gastroesophageal reflux disease: a possible association. Oral Dis. 2007;13(6):581–5.
21. Wondimu B, Nemeth A, Modeer T. Oral health in liver transplant children administered cyclosporin A or tacrolimus. Int J Paediatr Dent. 2001;11(6):424–9.
22. Hong CH, Scobey MW, Napenas JJ, Brennan MT, Lockhart PB. Dental postoperative bleeding complications in patients with suspected and documented liver disease. Oral Dis. 2012;18(7):661–6.
23. Tripodi A, Mannucci PM. The coagulopathy of chronic liver disease. N Engl J Med. 2011;365(2):147–56.
24. Medina JB, Andrade NS, de Paula Eduardo F, Bezinelli L, Franco JB, Gallottini M, et al. Bleeding during and after dental extractions in patients with liver cirrhosis. Int J Oral Maxillofac Surg. 2018;47(12):1543–9.
25. DeAngelis GA, Khot R, Haskal ZJ, Maitland HS, Northup PG, Shah NL, et al. Bleeding risk and management in interventional procedures in chronic liver disease. J Vasc Interv Radiol. 2016;27(11):1665–74.
26. Harrison MF. The misunderstood coagulopathy of liver disease: a review for the acute setting. West J Emerg Med. 2018;19(5):863–71.

27. Haghighi AG, Finder RG, Bennett JD. Systemic disease and bleeding disorders for the oral and maxillofacial surgeon. Oral Maxillofac Surg Clin N Am. 2016;28(4):461–71.
28. Prasanthi B, Kannan N, Patil R. Effect of diuretics on salivary flow, composition and oral health status: a clinico-biochemical study. Ann Med Health Sci Res. 2014;4(4):549–53.
29. Adegboyega T, Rivadeneira D. Lower GI bleeding: an update on incidences and causes. Clin Colon Rectal Surg. 2020;33(1):28–34.

Assessment of the Musculoskeletal System

9

William Conaway and William Hennrikus

9.1 Introduction

A familiarity with the brief musculoskeletal examination is critically important for any medical provider. Many subtle presentations can be indicative of underlying disease. Early management in musculoskeletal diseases and growth disorders can lead to less invasive and more successful outcomes. Recognition of some components of a patient's history and physical may be essential to avoiding complications during dental treatment.

9.2 Family History or Previous Medical History

It is not uncommon for children to have existing orthopedic diagnoses. Some diagnoses, such as cerebral palsy, arthrogryposis, or severe scoliosis, may make patient positioning difficult for dental examination and treatment. Other diagnoses, particularly those that involve instability of the cervical spine, may make positioning dangerous to the patient, e.g., Down syndrome. It is important to ask about issues with mobility of the joints, pain in the extremities or axial skeleton, or history of difficulty with weight bearing. It is also prudent to ask about a history of fractures because a child who is prone to fracture resulting from low-energy trauma may need to be screened for inborn or acquired pathology in bone formation such as osteogenesis imperfecta.

W. Conaway (✉)
Thomas Jefferson University, Philadelphia, PA, USA

W. Hennrikus
Department of Orthopaedics and Rehabilitation, Penn State College of Medicine, Hershey, PA, USA

9.3   Examination

9.3.1   Skin

Overall appearance of the skin should be noted. Café au lait spots or ash leaf spots can be indicative of systemic diseases including neurofibromatosis or tuberous sclerosis.

9.3.2   Neck

Range of motion of the neck should be assessed by rotating the child's head so the chin nearly points toward each shoulder, then by bending the neck so each ear nearly touches each shoulder, and then by flexing and extending the neck. Limited range of motion in the neck should warrant an orthopedic consult. In the young child, an abnormal range of motion of the cervical spine may be indicative of a congenital torticollis or possibly Klippel-Feil syndrome, each of which may complicate dental positioning.

9.3.3   Shoulders and Elbows

The range of motion of these joints should be tested by bringing the arm from the patient's side to above their head while also flexing and extending the elbow. Limited range of motion of these joints may be indicative of arthrogryposis. Typically, this will present with the shoulder in fixed internal rotation and the elbow fully extended without and elbow crease.

9.3.4   Hands and Forearms

Examination of the hands begins with an evaluation of the number and appearance of the fingers and thumbs. Polydactyly or syndactyly is often noted by caretakers prior to evaluation but can be subtle. Hypoplasia of any element of the hand, wrist, or forearm should be noted. A multitude of congenital hand/forearm conditions exist including Poland syndrome, cleft hand, radial club hand, thumb hypoplasia, and Madelung's deformity, all of which require orthopedic follow-up.

Passive range of motion of the fingers and wrist should also be evaluated. In particular, limited range of motion of the wrist with fixed flexed fingers and thumbs in adduction should raise concern for arthrogryposis or cerebral palsy. Very young children may be unable to extend their thumb which could indicate congenital trigger thumb [1].

Active range of motion of the upper extremity should be evaluated in young children, particularly those with a history of traumatic birth. Erb's palsy and Klumpke's palsy are caused by stretching of the brachial plexus and its roots at the cervical spine during delivery. These present with lack of ability to perform specific movements with the shoulder, elbow, wrist, and fingers and often a fixed posture due to this inability.

9.3.5 Knees and Legs

Any leg length discrepancy in the newborn should warrant an orthopedic consult.

Range of motion of the knees should be evaluated because lack of motion at this joint in a young child can be associated with arthrogryposis. This is generally apparent in the ambulatory child as contractures of the knee generally lead to significantly altered gait. Bowing of the legs should also be noted as this could be indicative of several underlying diagnoses such as neurofibromatosis or rickets.

9.3.6 Feet

Assessment of the feet should begin with evaluation of the number and appearance of the toes. Any additional digits, webbed digits, or hypoplasia of the foot or toes should warrant an orthopedic consultation. Two very common congenital deformities of the foot are metatarsus adductus and clubfoot deformity. Timely diagnosis can greatly impact treatment outcomes.

9.3.7 Spine

Examination of the spine should assess for symmetry of the shoulders, rib prominences, and flank prominences. Any lack of symmetry at any age until skeletal maturity should warrant an orthopedic consult for the evaluation of scoliosis. Scoliosis can be of idiopathic origin or can indicate an underlying diagnosis. Timely management of some forms of scoliosis can help avoid operative treatment.

9.3.8 Gait

Observation of the child's gait is essential to the orthopedic screening exam. The overall alignment of the lower limbs should be appreciated. In-toeing is often very concerning to caregivers but is most often physiologic under the age of 4. In older children it may warrant further evaluation. Bowed legs or genu varum is physiologic under the age of 2 but may represent a growth deformity known as infantile Blount's disease in children age 2–5. Bilateral knocked knees or genu valgum is physiologic under the age of 7 but over this age may represent deformity or even underlying disease such as renal osteodystrophy or a skeletal dysplasia.

A limp during examination always warrants further investigation and consultation. With a history of recent trauma, this could represent a fracture even in the absence of gross deformity. Toddler's fractures are subtle, minimally displaced spiral fractures of the tibia that occurs in children <2.5 years old. In similar age children without a history of trauma, there is concern for septic arthritis of the hip or toxic synovitis of the hip. These may require urgent surgical management, and as such the limping young child should be urgently evaluated. School-age children are at risk of the development of collapse of the femoral head known as Legg–Calve–Perthes disease. In the adolescent age group, new onset of limping with or without trauma should initiate investigation of slipped capital femoral epiphysis or other derangements of the bones, joints, or soft tissues of the lower extremities.

9.4 Orthopedic Findings/Diagnoses and How to Proceed

Congenital torticollis is a persistent painless head tilt or turn to one side due to a contracture of the sternocleidomastoid (SCM) muscle on one side. A palpable mass can be felt at the location of the SCM on one side. This condition is thought to be the result of an intrauterine packaging disorder and is treated in different ways at different ages. Risk factors for the disease include oligohydramnios, first pregnancy, traumatic delivery, and breech delivery, and associated conditions include developmental dysplasia of the hip and metatarsus adductus. These patients require orthopedic consultation prior to dental work in order to rule out occasionally associated cervical instability. Additionally, positioning for dental work may be complicated by the position of the neck.

Klippel-Feil syndrome is a rare congenital condition that causes failure of normal segmentation of the cervical spine during development. Features vary but can include partial cervical fusions and instability about the cervical spine that may preclude positioning for dental work without special anesthesia and positioning considerations.

Arthrogryposis is a congenital disorder of unknown etiology that presents with contractures and limited range of motion of multiple joints throughout the body. This condition may make positioning of the patient difficult, and the patient should be seen by an orthopedist for ongoing dental management.

Osteogenesis imperfecta is a genetic disorder that results from a mutation in the COL1A1 or COL1A2 genes leading to a decrease in type 1 collagen and poor collagen crosslinking. This results in unusually fragile bony structures and often presents with a history of multiple fractures from low-energy traumas.

Cerebral palsy is a congenital disorder caused by anoxic injury to the developing central nervous system that presents with cognitive and musculoskeletal expressions of widely varying severity. The neurologic injury is not progressive, but the musculoskeletal sequelae often are. Presentations vary widely and can include joint contractures, upper extremity deformity, spinal deformity, hip subluxation/dislocation, foot deformities, and gait disorders. Body positioning may make dental work challenging without general anesthesia.

Poland syndrome is a congenital disorder characterized by unilateral chest wall hypoplasia due to the absence of a portion of the pectoralis major muscle and symbrachydactyly of the ipsilateral hand. No special positioning was required.

Erb's palsy is an obstetric brachia plexopathy, i.e., injury to the brachial plexus, specifically the C5–C6 nerve roots that result in paralysis of the deltoid and biceps. The patient typically assumes a specific posture with the shoulder internally rotated at the patient's side, elbow extended, and wrist flexed. No special positioning was required.

Klumpke's palsy is an obstetric brachia plexopathy, i.e., injury to the brachial plexus, specifically the C8–T1 nerve roots that result in the development of a claw hand. No special positioning was required.

Neurofibromatosis is an autosomal dominant disorder caused by mutation of the NF1 gene that presents with skin lesions in addition to musculoskeletal involvement. Specifically, this can present as scoliosis, anterolateral bowing of the tibia, and deformities of the forearm. No special positioning was required.

Reference

1. Flynn, John M. M.D., and Stuart Weinstein M.D. Lovell and Winter's Pediatric Orthopaedics. 8th ed., LWW, 2020.

Assessment of the Brain

John Unkel

10.1 Overview of Neurologic History and Physical

Conditions effecting the nervous system can be complex leading to a variety of effects such as cognitive, sensory, motor, and reflexive disturbances. Due to this complexity, the content of the topics herein will be structured toward priorities of importance to the pediatric dentist. Similar to assessment of other systems, the neurologic evaluation begins with history taking. Grade-school guardians are usually the foremost providers of the initial chief complaint, after which time older children contribute to the history of the neurological concern. It is important to remember how the neurological concern fits into the normal developmental stages of the child, e.g., using three words in a sentence is anticipated for a 3-year-old, but not that of a 9-month-old.

A complete history is crucial to a neurological evaluation. Following the chief complaint, the neurologic history of present illness (HPI) begins with a symptomatic timeline of the concern. The HPI consists of anatomic location of concern, quality (e.g., achy, stabbing, etc.) and quantity/severity (e.g., graded scale where 1 = least pain and 10 = worst pain ever, or a faces scale, e.g., Wong-Baker) of the issue, timing, including onset, frequency and duration, environment situation occurred, factors alleviating and aggravating the concern, and associated symptoms/features. Birth history may be important for conditions that have been present for some time. The provider inquiring about the history of the child from birth gives the guardians confidence that the dentist desires to know about the entire medical history of the child which may be contributing to the chief complaint of a child with a chronic condition. With exception to precise developmental history, guardians generally provide an accurate history for children who are born healthy and progresses normally; however, prenatal/pregnancy, birth, and newborn issues may require

J. Unkel (✉)
Bon Secours Mercy Health System, St Mary's Hospital of Richmond, Richmond, VA, USA
e-mail: John_Unkel@bshsi.org

attainment of medical records for a complete history. Often obtained dental office health histories and acquired medical histories do not match. A medical history and review of systems are helpful to understand the conditions that affect the child and the proposed treatment the pediatric dentist may consider for a condition. Obtaining a family history is helpful for genetic transmission and inquiring about social history and often leads to environmental information such as stressors, e.g., divorce or family member death, school performance, diet, or living conditions, e.g., peeling paint, smoking in the home, and lead. Finally, the dentist should have a good understanding of a child's developmental progression by age, which is beyond the scope of this chapter. A slowing, relapse, or cessation of accomplished skills affecting motor, language, cognition, and social interaction is of concern as this may be related to a degenerative disease such as Rett syndrome or a metabolic problem that is affecting the central nervous system.

The pediatric neurologic examination begins when the children enter the office. Dental chairs can be positioned above the floor at a height allowing small children to climb up and position themselves. Frequently following a guardian or office staff's permission, children ambulate toward the dental chair and position themselves on the chair which immediately permits the dentist to develop a general assessment of a child's cognitive and neuromotor ability or disability. If a small child refuses or can't ambulate or must be carried by the guardian, observe the interaction with the guardian to observe for any developmental disabilities.

Once the child is positioned on the chair, the pediatric dentist should make a general craniofacial assessment and be adept at identifying dysmorphic craniofacial features (e.g., cranial size, plagiocephaly, telecanthus or hypertelorism, facial palsy, etc.) that may have associated neurologic considerations. While dentists do not routinely make measurements of head circumference, which are routine by pediatricians for children up to age 2, general craniofacial irregularities should be noted and reported to the child's physician and craniofacial team where appropriate. Small skulls can represent lack of brain growth or fusion of cranial sutures. Conversely, a large head can be due to genetics, hydrocephalus, hemorrhage, etc. Pediatric dentists begin to evaluate children as early as 6 months and fontinales can be assessed. In young children up to about 18 months, the anterior fontanel is open and on palpation should be soft, flat, and pulsatile. Either absence of the anterior fontanel or a bulging fontanel is abnormal and should be further evaluated.

10.2 Mental Status

Begin a new patient craniofacial-oral examination of a child/adolescent in the upright chair position if possible. A slow deliberate approach speaking with the child and allowing the child to identify his/her anatomic structures (e.g., "show me your ear") is preferable rather than initially attempting to evaluate the oral cavity. This approach yields a more cooperative child/adolescent, leading to a better evaluation. Initially, a measure of facial expression, manner, affect, and relationship to the guardian, staff, and doctor can be assessed. Anxiety, irritation, flat affect, or developmental delay may be noted. The pediatric dentist can use play as a method to interact with young children, whereas with older children/adolescents, small talk about school may be a good starting point. Developmentally appropriate language is a good indicator of mental status after repour has been established. The recall of several objects or the child stating their person, place, and time are good starting points on consultations and comprehensive dental examinations for assessing orientation.

Children with clinical neurological manifestations affecting the craniofacial structures are frequently encountered by pediatric dentists. Two types of evaluations can be performed to assess altered mental status (AMS): (1) qualitative or (2) quantitative. Qualitative assessments are generally utilized more in the office or hospital setting for assessing level of consciousness and labeling pathologic processes, whereas the quantitative Glasgow Coma Scale (GCS) is frequently utilized for trauma when the dentist encounters a child with an altered level of consciousness suggesting a neurologic injury. The scale is modified for infants. The GCS allows a number to be assigned for each criterion: motor, verbal, and ocular. The scores for each of the three categories are added for a total score. A total score below 15 on GCS after a trauma should signify to the dentist that further workup is warranted.

AMS (five levels of consciousness)—Qualitative

Normal: awake, alert or arousable

Lethargic: in and out of alert state

Obtunded: reduction in level of alertness, response to pain, and other stimuli

Stuporous: responds to pain only

Comatose: unresponsive

AMS Glasgow Coma Scale—Quantitative

Motor	6	follows commands
	5	Localizes pain
	4	Withdraws from pain
	3	Abnormal flexion to pain (decorticate)
	2	Abnormal extension to pain (decerebrate)
	1	Flaccid
Verbal	5	Oriented
	4	Confused
	3	Inappropriate vocabulary
	2	Unrecognizable sounds
	1	Nonverbal
Eyes	4	Open spontaneously
	3	Open to sound
	2	Open to pain
	1	Does not open eyes

10.3   Cranial Nerves

There are 12 (I–XII) cranial nerves that are part of the peripheral nervous system although the olfactory (I) and optic (II) nerves are actually nerve fiber tracts directly from the brain.

Olfactory nerve (I). CNI is a special visceral afferent nerve providing the sense of smell that extends from the nasal olfactory nerve fibers through the cribriform plate of the ethmoid bone to the olfactory bulb and brain. The sense of smell can be affected by trauma to the nerve passing through a fractured cribriform plate or infection, which may lead to inflammation of the nasal epithelium, olfactory stem cells, or rarely the nerve/nerve fibers themselves leading to anosmia or hyposmia. Sense of smell can be tested by occluding on nostril and passing a common smelling substance under the open nostril and asking the patient for a response to the stimulus. Then repeat the procedure with the opposite nostril. On a conscious patient, it is preferable to avoid noxious substances such as ammonia inhalants as they also may stimulate CNV, thus not isolating response to CNI.

Optic and oculomotor nerves (II–III). CNII is a special somatic afferent nerve that provides vision. Visual acuity or visual sharpness is grossly measured by a Snellen eye chart (pediatric Allen chart for toddlers). An ideal 20/20 vision determines how well an individual positioned 20 ft. can read the chart. The top number refers to the distance of 20 ft. For instance, an individual with a 20/30 vision can read the Snellen chart letters at 20 ft. that most people can interpret at 30 feet. Conversely, a 20/15 vision means that a person can see at 20 feet what most people see at 15 feet. A visual field is the area seen by an eye when the individual focuses on a distant object or point. The total visual field is divided into nasal (closest to the nose) and lateral temporal fields. Fields are further divided into upper and lower quadrants. The total visual field of both eyes has overlapping binocular vision centrally and monocular vision laterally. Fields can be screened by having the patient close one eye and the clinician putting one hand behind each ear several feet from the head and then wiggling the fingers of each hand moving forward to the patient's center of vision. A toy or other colored objects can be used for young children. The patient should notify the dentist as soon as the fingers/object in each hand become visible. All four quadrants should be tested. Any field defect should be referred for further evaluation. Defects can be due to optic neuritis/neuropathy, optic chiasm/pituitary tumors, stroke, etc. Pupils should be checked for size, shape, position, and reactivity. Reactivity depends on stimulation of the optic nerve and its connection to CNIII in the midbrain which then stimulates the iris sphincter and ciliary muscles. The pupillary reaction (constriction or dilatation) is observed by the swinging light test. Light stimulates the optic nerve, and the stimulus travels to the midbrain to stimulate the general visceral efferent portion of CNIII leading to pupillary constriction. Direct reaction is constriction in the pupil in which the light is flashed and consensual constriction occurs simultaneously in the opposing eye pupil. Dim the room light and ask the patient to focus on a distant object in the room. Shine the light in one eye for a few seconds and then the other watching for the direct and consensual constriction of the pupils. Acute anisocoria from unilateral mydriasis or "blown pupil" following head trauma may be due to brain herniation and increased intracranial pressure affecting CNIII or due to an anticholinergic chemical in the eye such atropine. Chronic unilateral pupillary constriction may be due to sympathetic pathway pathology resulting in Horner syndrome (meiosis, ptosis, and anhidrosis). In cases of trauma and chemical stimulation, the affected pupil will be unresponsive, whereas in Horner syndrome, the affected pupil may be slow to dilate (dilatation lag) in a dimly lit room but be responsive to direct light.

Oculomotor, trochlear, and abducent nerves (CNIII, IV, and VI). CNIII, IV, and VI are general somatic efferent nerves for extraocular eye movement. CNIII activates the three rectus (medial, superior, and inferior) muscles, which adducts, elevates, and depresses the globe as well as the inferior oblique that elevates and abducts the globe. Lastly, the nerve elevates the upper eyelid via the levator palpebrae muscle. An epidural or subdural hematoma following a trauma can lead to paralysis of the nerve causing downward and lateral movement of the globe, ptosis, and diplopia. CN IV moves the eye down and in. This nerve travels around the midbrain and decussates in the area of the brainstem at the superior medullary velum, and trauma can result in bilateral nerve palsies due to extortion and elevation of the eye. CN VI abducts the eye toward the lateral commissure. Paralysis of the nerve due to trauma, meningitis, or increased intracranial pressure results in medial deviation of the eye and horizontal double vision. These three motor nerves can be tested by the examiner moving a finger in the six cardinal directions of gaze—an "H" movement. Disconjugate eye gaze, defined as, failure of both eyes to align in the same horizontal and vertical planes during anesthesia traditionally, has been noted to occur during stage 2 anesthesia. However, recent findings suggest that unlike clinical signs of body movement, cough, and grimace, which occur generally sequentially with discontinuance of sevoflurane, disconjugate gaze does not occur as part of a systematic pattern. Disconjugate gaze can also be observed during levels of sedation. Administration of sedative and anesthetics likely affects the motor nuclei that control eye movements.

Trigeminal nerve (CN V). The dentist is very familiar with this nerve and its three branches: ophthalmic V-1, maxillary V-2, and mandibular V-3. The special visceral efferent V-3 branch innervates and provides motor ability to the muscles of mastication (temporalis, masseter, and pterygoids) as well as the tensor tympani, mylohyoid, and anterior digastric. Palsy of this branch results in flaccid paralysis of the muscles of mastication with deviation of the mandible to the side of the paralysis and difficulty moving the jaw in the opposite direction. Paralysis of the tensor tympani results in inability to hear low pitch tones. The general somatic efferent branches of V1–3 provide sensation to the skin of the upper, middle, and lower face, mucosa of the mouth, nose and frontal and maxillary sinuses, and lacrimal glands and are responsible for the corneal reflex. Each branch of the nerve should be tested if damage is suspected: V-1 corneal reflex should show blinking of each eye and sensitivity of the forehead, bridge of nose, and philtrum skin and V2–3 acknowledgement of sensation by touching both sides of the mid and lower face for verification of sensation bilaterally.

Facial nerve (CN VII). CN VII is a complex nerve with general sensory, special sensory, parasympathetic properties, and motor function. The limited spectrum of the general somatic afferent fibers provides sensation by innervating the posterior surface of the auricle and external auditory canal. The general visceral afferent fibers provide sensation to the soft palate and pharyngeal wall. The special visceral afferent fibers of the chorda tympani provide taste in the anterior two thirds of the tongue. It can be tested by placing a salty or sour substance on each side of the tongue. The general visceral efferent components stimulate submandibular and sublingual saliva and lacrimal tear release. Finally, the special visceral efferent fibers innervate the muscles of facial expression, platysma, stapedius, stylohyoid, and posterior belly of the digastric. The upper facial muscles (forehead) are innervated ipsilaterally, and the lower face is innervated by the contralateral nerve. Hence, an upper motor neuron lesion of the brain primarily causes flaccidity in the lower face on the opposite side, and a lower peripheral motor nerve lesion, e.g., Bell's palsy by Lyme disease or herpes virus, causes flaccidity to upper and lower portions of the face on the same side as the nerve lesion. The upper nerve can be tested by raising the eyebrows and the face in general by closing the eyes, frowning, puffing out cheeks, and smiling.

Vestibulocochlear nerve (CNVIII). CN VIII is a special sensory afferent nerve with two portions: vestibular and cochlear. The vestibular portion maintains equilibrium, balance, and orientation in space, whereas the cochlear portion is for hearing. A common patient complaint with vestibular dysfunction is that the room is spinning or a feeling of rotation (vertigo). Patients may be noticed to have nystagmus with the fast motion of movement away from the side of the head of the injured nerve. When the patient stands with feet together and then closes the eyes for 30–60 s, the individual may lose balance and lean/fall toward the effected ear (positive Romberg test). The cochlear branch is easily tested in the dental office by the whisper test for hearing. The dentist can stand behind the patient's chair in the upright position, cover one ear, and whisper a few words or rub fingers to test the uncovered ear for hearing by having the child repeat back the words (most sensitive) or confirm a rubbing sound. These procedures can be repeated for the other ear. Detected hearing loss can be conductive (externa auditory canal and middle ear) or sensorineural (inner ear), and if detected, the child is to be referred to audiology and otolaryngology (ENT) for distinction. Hearing is crucial for language development, especially during the first 3 years of life. Early hearing detection and intervention involves a screening test that is usually done by the hospital before discharge of a newborn. If an irregularity is detected, the baby will need to follow up with an audiologist and ENT for further comprehensive evaluation. Common congenital reasons for hearing loss include infections (e.g., TORCHES, medications, hypoxia, prematurity with NICU stay, or a genetic reason, e.g., CHARGE). Late hearing loss can be due to genetic/syndrome causes or a virus.

Glossopharyngeal and vagus nerves (CN IX and X). CN IX is primarily a sensory nerve where the dentist is concerned, whereas X has sensory components but is primarily motor in the head and neck. The CN IX provides general somatic components, which innervates the external ear, auditory canal, and tympanic membrane, whereas the general visceral components provide sensation to the posterior tongue and pharynx that can lead to a gag reflex and also innervates the carotid sinus baroreceptors and carotid body chemoreceptors. Baroreceptors and chemoreceptors are critical to monitoring blood pressure and pH, pO_2, and PCO_2, which are key during sedation. The posterior taste buds are innervated by the special visceral efferent component, which can affect detection of bitter substances. The parotid gland is innervated by a parasympathetic component, leading to saliva production. Damage to the nerve by ischemia, retropharyngeal abscesses, or masses can lead to loss of gag reflex, loss of taste, or syncope (carotid sinus). The CN X component that interests dentists are the special efferent components. The special visceral efferent portion provides motor innervation to the uvula, pharynx, larynx (gag reflex), and esophagus except for the stylopharyngeus and tensor palatini muscles. The general visceral efferent is responsible for parasympathetic activities in the neck, heart, lungs, and abdomen. Injury to the nerve can lead to loss of gag reflex and ipsilateral paralysis of soft palate, which may lead to inferior positioning, hoarse voice, impaired cough reflex, difficulty swallowing, and vocal cord paralysis. The nerves can be tested by having the patient say "Ah" looking for symmetrical elevation and medial movement of the soft palate toward the uvula in the midline. Touching each side of the pharynx can test the gag reflex by looking for unilateral differences.

Accessory nerve (CN XI): CN XI is a special visceral motor nerve that innervates the sternocleidomastoid and trapezius muscles. The nerves permit rotating the head contralaterally and flexing the neck and elevates the shoulders respectively. If damaged, paralysis of the muscles leading to limited head rotation and flexion and shoulder drooping is noticed. Fasciculations and atrophy of the trapezius muscle and winging of the scapula may be noticed if the nerve is affected. The trapezius is tested by superiorly shrugging the shoulders and the sternocleidomastoid by rotating the head against a hand on the opposite side of the chin, resisting the movement or raising the head off a flat surface.

Hypoglossal nerve (CNXII). CN XII permits tongue movement. This general somatic efferent nerve innervates both muscles of tongue and extrinsic muscles (genioglossus, styloglossus, and hyoglossus). Paralysis of one side causes protrusion toward the injured side of the tongue or affected nerve. If the tongue is affected, bilaterally swallowing and total tongue protrusion are limited. Fasciculations of the tongue and inability to push tongue against cheek may be noted with an injured nerve. Injuries or congenital anomalies in the area of the foramen magnum can lead to CN XII malfunction.

10.4 Motor Evaluation

Children ambulating toward the dental chair and then climbing up into the chair and positioning in the chair can provide the dentist critical information. It's important to distinguish gait orthopedic limitations from neurologic limitations such as hemiparesis and cerebral palsy; a good medical history and positioning of the child comfortably on the chair are essential in these instances. Once positioned the dentist should look for involuntary movements such as tics; fasciculations, especially of the tongue; dystonia; tremors; and chorea.

Bulk: Increased muscle bulk leading to hypertrophy is related to normal use/exercise or excessive parafunctional use that the dentist may notice bilaterally on the face from excessive masseter muscle activity due to clenching or grinding. Pseudohypertrophy results from muscle being replaced with other tissues leading to limitation of movement or weakness. An example is Duchenne muscular dystrophy. Children affected with Duchenne have proximal muscle weakness and often position themselves in a tripod when rising from the floor using other muscles in addition to those in the legs to rise from the floor (Gowers sign). Atrophy can result from muscle disuse or neurologic injury or disease.

Tone: Tone can be considered as overall muscle stiffness or resistance to active or passive stretch, but the muscles at rest have a certain amount of tension. Irregularities of tone include hypotonia, rigidity, and spasticity. Hypotonia can be flaccidity, which occurs with pathology/damage to the central or peripheral nervous systems and muscle or neuromuscular junction. An infant with Prader-Willi syndrome is an example. Rigidity can be considered resistance to flexion or extension that is not rate dependent and can be due to pathology of the basal ganglia. Finally, spasticity is due to upper motor neuron pathology and is considered rate dependent rigidity detected toward the ends of the range of motion. Children with cerebral palsy may have the spastic form of the disease. Tone may be checked by holding the child's hands in yours and passively moving their hands, elbows, and shoulders to check for resistance.

Strength and coordination: Children love to show how active they can be. Children jumping up and down, making a muscle, and squeezing the dentist's hands are good tests. Strength is graded from 0 (none) to 5 (normal) and full resistance without fatigue. Notice the child's movements when walking toward the chair for lack of coordination or ataxia. If the gait seems unusual, ask about cerebellar pathology, and if none is recalled by the guardian, have the child walk and maintain a heel to toe line if of the appropriate age to check for coordination. The upper extremity can be evaluated by having the child's index finger touch your outstretched fingers pointing toward him/her and then have the child touch his/her nose. This further test cerebellar function.

10.5 Sensory Examination

This was previously discussed with the cranial nerves which is relevant to dentistry. The nerves should be tested bilaterally by touching each side of the face, tongue, ear, etc.

10.5.1 Reflexes

Deep tendon reflexes consist of the triceps, biceps, brachioradialis, knee, and ankle. Grading the reflex ranges from 0 (no response) to 4+ (hyperactive) with 2 considered as normal. Hypoactive reflexes are generally due to lower motor pathology or cerebellar deficit, whereas hyperactive responses are attributed to upper motor neurons. Children with cerebral palsy may be hyper-reflexive. The jaw jerk (masseter) reflex is a stretch reflex used to test injury to the *trigeminal nerve* (CNV). The chin is tapped with the mouth slightly open in a downward angle. Without trigeminal injury very little, if any, upward jerk of the mandible will be present. However, with upper motor neuron lesions above the foramen magnum, an accentuated upward jerk will be present.

10.5.2 Common Neurological Conditions of Interest to the Dentist

Neurofibromatosis is an autosomal dominant inherited disorder and NF-1 is attributed to chromosome 17q and NF-2 chromosome 22 and both can occur spontaneously. The syndrome consists of two types: NF-1 and NF-2. NF-1 should have at least two of seven classic characteristics: (1) six or more café-au-lait spots larger than 5 mm in greatest diameter in prepubertal children and greater than 15 mm in post-pubertal children with a smooth coast of California border (as opposed to McCune-Albright syndrome irregular coast of Maine and basal cell nevus syndrome), (2) two or more neurofibromas of any type or one plexiform neurofibroma, (3) axillary or inguinal freckling, (4) two or more Lisch nodules, (5) optic glioma, (6) osseous lesions (e.g., sphenoid dysplasia leading to exophthalmos), and (7) a first degree relative with NF-1. These children additionally may suffer from learning disabilities, seizures, cerebral vascular malformations, and cancers. Careful head and neck exams for rhabdomyosarcomas and blood pressure monitoring for hypertension, possibly due to pheochromocytoma, are essential. Oral abnormalities are associated with plexiform neurofibromas from the trigeminal nerve. Commonly, neurofibromas are common on the tongue and occasionally on the oral mucosa and gingiva. Bony changes include increased dimension of the coronoid notch, deformity of the condylar head, and an enlarged mandibular foramen. NF-2 is primarily due to schwannomas/neuromas primarily on CN VIII, but also CN VII, which affect hearing and balance and lead to tinnitus and facial weakness.

Tuberous sclerosis is an autosomal dominant disorder that has a high spontaneous occurrence due to errors on 9q coding for tumor suppressor protein hamartin and the 16p chromosome coding for tumor suppressor protein tuberin. The loss of either protein leads to hamartomas (benign tumors). The condition affects the skin, brain, heart, kidneys, and lung and has oral manifestations. Oral findings include fibromas affecting the gingiva, tongue mucosa, lips, and tooth enamel pitting along with more common major skin (angiofibromas, ash-leaf spots, Shagreen patches) findings, cortical tubers, subependymal nodules of the lateral ventricles, and periungual fibromas. These children often have seizures, developmental delay, and autism spectrum disorders. Subependymal nodules require monitoring with MRI scans as they can develop into subependymal giant cell astrocytomas.

Sturge-Weber syndrome is a vascular disorder following the trigeminal nerve (always ophthalmic division) caused by mutation of the GNAQ gene, which encodes G-protein alpha q leading to enlargement of capillaries of the face, maxilla, and blood vessels of the brain meninges and eye, resulting in the facial port-wine stain, and affects neurotransmitters. Seizures, hemiparesis, developmental delay, and headaches are findings in these children. CT scans frequently show calcifications of the brain. The vascular abnormalities may affect the oral gingiva, floor of the mouth, cheeks, palate, lips, and pharyngeal mucosa. Clinical planning must be undertaken with multidisciplinary specialists when invasive oral procedures and local anesthesia delivery are considered due to bleeding risk.

Cerebral palsy is a disorder of motor impairment affecting movement and positioning due to anomalies of the brain such as preterm infantile intracerebral hemorrhage and periventricular leukomalacia. These children often have behavioral, sensory, cognitive, and communicative impairment. Common classifications include spastic (most common affecting motor cortex), dyskinetic (basal ganglia), and ataxic (cerebellum) cerebral palsy which further can be broken down into quadriplegia, hemiplegia, and diplegia. Sedation of these children can be challenging due to gastroesophageal reflux, poor protective laryngeal and pharyngeal reflexes, and a higher bispectral index score suggesting they achieve a higher level of sedation with a routine sedative dose of a medication. Opioids have shown a greater potency but increase the risk for respiratory depression. Children with cerebral palsy may have difficulty swallowing, impaired coughing, and increased salivary gland secretion, creating a risk for aspiration. Positioning patients in the dental chair may not be optimal due to contractures and/or scoliosis.

Autism spectrum disorder is a neurodevelopmental disability consisting of limitations in communication and social interaction. The disability is further distinguished by behavior disorders, including repetitive actions, obsession pertaining to redundant patterns, aggression, focused attention on limited interests, and restricted activities, and individuals can be afflicted by seizure activity. Autism affects the cerebellum and limbic system beginning in infancy and proceeds into adulthood. Sensory perceptions and deficits affect the visual, auditory, olfactory, tactile, and gustatory processing functions. A narrow group of autistic children with macrocephaly have been identified with a mutated PTEN gene. Oral health tends to be worse in these individuals due to preference for sweetened foods and pouching and retaining these foods due to impaired tongue coordination leading to caries. Due to behavioral aberrancies, this population of children can resist accommodation to dental procedures to improve oral health and require sedation or general anesthesia. However, these children can be difficult to sedate for stimulating procedures. Recently successful sedative approaches frequently utilize dexmedetomidine alone due to its neuroprotective effects or with nitrous oxide or midazolam for imaging, auditory brainstem response testing, and dental procedures. For painful procedures emergency rooms commonly employ ketamine. Pediatric patients with neurologic disorders and developmental disabilities who are administered sedation can be at risk for adverse airway and impaired respiratory mechanics. Recovery from sedation can be challenging as these children become agitated awaking in a nonfamiliar environment and can injure themselves or others. Guardians may be beneficial to have present to smooth recovery as the child will have someone known to them and feel more secure.

Chiari (Arnold-Chiari) malformation is an inferior brain anomaly where the cerebellum and brainstem are positioned below the foreman magnum (type I) and with a corresponding myelomeningocele (type II) or where the cerebellum and brainstem are displaced through a posterior skull defect (III). Type I individuals may not be aware they have the defect until it becomes symptomatic later in life due to dysfunction of lower cranial nerves, apnea, alteration in gait, headache, vertigo, and/or neck discomfort. Extremity spasticity or weakness or bowel and bladder dysfunction suggest developing spinal cord involvement. Type II typically appears during early infancy or early childhood and is associated with myelomeningocele and hydrocephalus. Symptoms are similar to type I, e.g., lower cranial nerve defects are common with the addition of partial paralysis below the associated spina bifida defect. Type III is diagnosed at birth and is associated with debilitating and life-threatening events. These children have symptoms similar to type II but additionally have association with seizures and developmental delays. Dental specialists may be consulted due to trigeminal neuralgia and referred pain to the temporomandibular joint and masseter muscles due to intracranial pressure that affects the trigeminal tract that parallels the spinal cord.

Further Reading

Ammari MM, Ribeiro P, de Souza I, Maia LC, Primo LG. Oral findings in a family with tuberous sclerosis complex. Spec Care Dentist. 2015;35(5):261–5.

Bardellini E, Amadori F, Flocchini P, Conti G, Piana G, Majorana A. Oral findings in 50 children with neurofibromatosis type 1: a case control study. Eur J Paediatr Dent. 2011;12(4):256–60.

Bennett J, Pelak V. Palsies of the third, fourth, and sixth cranial nerves. Neuro-Ophthalmology. 2001;14(1):169–83.

Bickley LS, Szilagyi PG. Bates guide to physical examination and history taking. 12th ed. Philadelphia: Wolters Kluwer; 2017. p. 736–45.

Brown JJ, Gray JM, Roback MG, Sethuraman U, Farooqi A, Kannikeswaran N. Procedural sedation in children with autism spectrum disorders in the emergency department. Am J Emerg Med. 2019;37:1404–8.

Burton LJ, Kamat PP. The pediatric procedural sedation handbook. New York: Oxford University Press; 2018. p. 200–7.

Cornelissen L, Donado C, Lee LM, Liang NE, Mills I, Tou A, Aykut B, Berde CB. Clinical signs and electroencephalographic patterns of emergence from sevoflurane anesthesia in children: an observational study. Eur J Anaesthesiol. 2018;35:49–59.

De Arruda J, Figueiredo E, Monteiro J, Barbosa L, Rodriguez C, Vasconcelos B. Orofacial clinical features in Arnold Chiairi type 1 malformation: a case series. J Exp Dent. 2018;10(4):378–82.

Ferranzzano GF, Salerno C, Bravaccio C, Ingenito A, Sangianatoni G, Cantile T. Autism spectrum disorders and oral health status: a review of the literature. Eur J Paediatr Dent. 2020;21(1):9–12.

Fix JD. High yield neuroanatomy. 3rd ed. Philadelphia: Lippincott Williams & Wilkins; 2005. p. 89–102.

Herrera-Moncada M, Campos-Lara P, Hernandez-Cabanillas JC, Bermeo-Escalona JR, Pozos-Guillen A, Pozos-Guillen F, Garrocho-Rangel JA. Autism and paediatric dentistry: a scoping review. Oral Health Prev Dent. 2018;17(3):203–10.

Kilbaugh TJ, Friess SH, Raghupathi R, Huh JW. Sedation and analgesia in children with developmental disabilities and neurologic disorders. Int J Pediatr. 2010;2010:189142.

Kovalesky MB, Unkel JH, Reinhartz J, Reinhartz D. Discrepancies between dental parent-derived health histories and medical electronic records. Pediatr Dent. 2019;41(5):371–5.

Leyman RK, Schor NF. Neurologic evaluation. In: Nelson textbook of pediatrics. 20th ed. Philadelphia: Elsevier; 2016. p. 2791–817.

Li BL, Yuen VM, Zhang N, Zhang HH, Huang JX, Yang SY. A comparison of intranasal dexmedetomidine plus buccal midazolam for non-painful procedure sedation in children with autism. J Dev Disord. 2019;49:3798–806.

Lieu J, Kenna M, Anne S, Davidson L. Hearing loss in children a review. JAMA. 2021;324(21):2195–205.

Lubisch N, Roskos R, Berkenbosch JW. Dexmedetomidine for procedural sedation in children with autism and other behavioral disorders. Pediatr Neurol. 2009;41:88–94.

Mangione F, Bdeoui F, Monnier-Da Costa A, Dursun E. Autistic patients: a retrospective study on their dental needs and behavioral approach. Clin Oral Investig. 2020;24:1677–85.

Martins ML, Letieri ADS, Lenzi MM, Agostini M, Castro GF. Oral healthcare management of a child with phakomatosis pigmentovascularis associated with bilateral Sturge-Weber syndrome. Special Care Dentist. 2019;39(3):324–9.

Patel S, Mutyala S, Leske D, Hodge D, Holmes J. Incidence, associations, and evaluation of sixth nerve palsy using a population-based method. J Ophthamol. 2004;111:369–75.

Reshef ER, Schiff ND, Brown EN. A neurologic examination for anesthesiologists. Anesthesiology. 2019;130(3):462–71.

Rowe F. Prevalence of ocular motor cranial nerve palsy and associations following stroke. Eye. 2011;25:881–7.

Unkel JH, Cruise C, Rice A, MacDonald J, Berry EJ, Reinhartz J, Reinhartz D. A retrospective evaluation of the safety profile of dexmedetomidine and nitrous oxide for pediatric dental sedation. J Pediatr Dent. 2021;34(2):129–32.

Varma R, Williams SD, Wessel HB. Atlas of pediatric physical diagnosis. 6th ed. Philadelphia: Elsevier Saunders; 2012. p. 585–94.

Assessment of the Teenager

11

S. Thikkurissy

The American Academy of Pediatrics defines adolescence as the chronologic ages between 11 and 21 [1]. It is important to note that this age span is defined by major physical, psychological, and emotional changes. The adolescent has monitoring needs and anticipatory guidance requirements that exceed younger children. These include questioning into use of illicit substances, as well as tobacco usage. Seventy one percent of teenagers reported at least one potential health risk, yet according to Chung et al., only 37% of these teenagers reported discussing any of these risks with their primary care physician [2]. Adolescents engage in more intentional risk-taking behaviors than younger populations. These include but are not limited to alcohol and drug use/abuse and at-risk sexual behaviors. Giedd has demonstrated that there is an overall increase in impulsivity in the developing adolescent brain. This is countered with the fact that Giedd also concluded: "White matter increases throughout adolescence, which allows the older adolescent and adult brain to conduct more complex cognitive tasks and adaptive behavior" [3]. While the medical history assessment is somewhat similar, these issues should be addressed as specifically as possible.

In a national survey from 1998, 29.5% of students reported that they had been pregnant or had gotten someone pregnant. Ethnic differences have been noted as well. Overall, black and Hispanic students (42.4% and 31.4%, respectively) were significantly more likely than white students (22.7%) to have been pregnant or gotten someone pregnant. Related to anesthesia and sedation, the American Society of Anesthesiologists (ASA) recommend "pregnancy testing may be offered to female patients of childbearing age and for whom the result would alter the patient's management. Informed consent or assent of the risks, benefits, and alternatives related to preoperative pregnancy testing should be obtained" [4]. Recommendations supported by the ASA include:

S. Thikkurissy (✉)
Cincinnati Children's Hospital, Cincinnati, OH, USA
e-mail: Sarat.thikkurissy@cchmc.org

89

S. Thikkurissy, S. Golkari (eds.), *History and Physical for the Pediatric Dental Patient*, https://doi.org/10.1007/978-3-031-51458-6_11

1. Pregnancy tests are not warranted in patients less than 13 years old, unless there is any evidence of active sexual history.
2. If the patient is 13 or older, or at least 1-year post-menses, a pregnancy test is recommended.
3. If the patient is getting a pregnancy test, a urine test is sufficient.

This may require that the adolescent be sent to their physician/pediatrician within 24 h of sedation for a pregnancy test and result.

It should be underscored that the AAP classification of adolescence mentioned earlier is a chronologic age-based classification. The provider must take care to review with family and potential for developmental delay and/or neurobehavioral diagnoses as included in the neurology chapter.

Another area to consider is the transgender/sexual dysmorphic patient. This population who are still in search of their sexual identity is increasing in prevalence. National studies tend to place the prevalence around 1%, but some studies have demonstrated prevalence as high as 2.3% [5, 6]. A 2017 article by Schwartz suggests strategies to make practices more inclusive; these include:

1. On intake forms, provide one selection for "Sex at Birth" and a separate free space to write "Gender Identity."
2. On intake forms, ask for "legal name" separately from "name."
3. Give patients choice and encourage to select posttreatment rewards (such as not giving all girls princesses and boys cars, etc.).
4. Use gender-neutral terminology. If uncertain, ask how patients prefer to be addressed.
5. Refrain making assumptions about sexual orientation based on outward appearance. For instance, Female Patient: I'm going to homecoming this weekend. Doctor: Who are you going with? (Avoid: Are you going with your boyfriend?)
6. Place a rainbow decal or button in the door or a visible bulletin board, which can be a sign of acceptance and comfort to families.

The adolescent patient presents another difference from the young child, which is the concept of assent. The adolescent while in many cases developmentally approaching adult maturity will not attain legal maturity until 18, yet their voice and acknowledgment in procedures being performed on their body are critical. According to Lind et al., gaining assent "demonstrates respect of the minor and of her or his autonomy, helps to promote the therapeutic alliance and relationship, helps to empower the minor on her or his own behalf, and communicates the message that the minor will be an active participant in her or his own treatment" [7]. While consent may have been obtained prior to the sedation appointment, reviewing and ensuring that the patient assents to treatment is important. Many institutions will use the chronologic age of 8 as a guidance for attaining assent. However, the provider should evaluate the developmental maturity of the patient, as assent may be beneficial in younger patients as well.

Another consideration for the pre-teen and teen patient is the use of illicit (and in some states legal) substances. Vaping is a popular trend which Bonner notes "is the process of inhaling and exhaling an aerosol produced by an e-cigarette, vape pen, or personal aerosolizer. When the device contains nicotine, the Food and Drug Administration (FDA) lists the product as an electronic nicotine delivery system or ENDS device. Similar electronic devices can be used to vape cannabis extracts." [8] A PubMed search reveals the term "vaping" produced 1108 publications in 2020. Much of the literature with regard to vaping deals with the potential for vaping-specific lung disease. Many of the vaping products still contain nicotine which carry the same potential for lung damage as cigarettes. These ENDS (electronic nicotine delivery system) products also have been noted for risk of toxicity from flavorings. Flavoring compounds have been identified as sources of toxicity from ENDS devices; however, compared to the hundreds of flavoring constituents found in e-liquids, there are relatively few studies addressing the specific flavoring chemicals driving ENDS toxicity [9]. These products can contribute to persistent low-grade inflammatory processes in both the pulmonary and cardiovascular system. Careful assessment should be undertaken, and if positive, a physician-directed H&P is requested to determine any deficit in lung function.

The adolescent patient is one who is undergoing physical, emotional, and psychological change. The sedating provider must be aware of this and include this into treatment planning the sedation.

References

1. Hagan JF, Shaw JS, Duncan PM, editors. Bright futures: guidelines for health supervision of infants, children, and adolescents. 4th ed. American Academy of Pediatrics: Elk Grove Village, IL; 2017.
2. Chung PJ, Lee TC, Morrison JL, Schuster MA. Preventive care for children in the United States: quality and barriers. Annu Rev Public Health. 2006;27:491–515.
3. Giedd JN. The teen brain: insights from neuroimaging. J Adolesc Health. 2008;42(4):335–43.
4. American Society of Anesthesiologists. Pregnancy testing prior to anesthesia and surgery committee of origin: quality management and departmental administration.
5. Agana MG, Greydanus DE, Indyk JA, et al. Caring for the transgender adolescent and young adult: current concepts of an evolving process in the 21st century. Dis Mon. 2019;65(9):303–56. https://doi.org/10.1016/j.disamonth.2019.07.004.
6. Zucker KJ. Epidemiology of gender dysphoria and transgender identity. Sex Health. 2017;14(5):404–11. https://doi.org/10.1071/SH17067.
7. Schwartz SLGBT. Let's go beyond teeth. Pediatr Dent. 2017;39(2):90–2.
8. Bonner E, Chang Y, et al. The chemistry and toxicology of vaping. Pharmacol Ther. 2021;225:107837.
9. Adams TB, Cohen SM, Doull J, V.J., et al. Extract manufacturers, a the FEMA GRAS assessment of benzyl derivatives used as flavor ingredients. Food Chem Toxicol. 2005;43:1207–40.

COVID-19 and Procedural Sedation

12

S. Thikkurissy

The introduction of, and subsequent pandemic-level spread of, the SARS-CoV-2 virus, known commonly as COVID-19, has impacted every aspect of modern life. The assessment of the patient for procedural sedation is no different. While rates of transmission, hospitalization, and chronic illness may vary from community to community, the dentist managing dental disease in this context needs some grounded means for assessment.

It should be stated at the outset, it is this author's recommendation that children with a positive history of symptomatic COVID-19 infection requiring supplemental oxygen therapy or hospitalization are not candidates for in-office procedural sedation. Reasons for this recommendation are forthcoming. The child we will discuss in this chapter will primarily be the child who has an incidental history of COVID-19 infection but either with no or minor systemic symptoms. According to Alsohime (2020), "The most commonly reported symptoms in children aged ≤9 years were fever (46%), cough (37%), headache (15%), diarrhea (14%), and sore throat (13%). In children aged 10–19 years, headache (42%), cough (41%), fever (35%), myalgia (30%), sore throat (29%), shortness of breath (16%), and diarrhea (14%) [1]. For the pediatric dentist, this compendium of symptoms overlaps with those of other common pediatric infectious diseases. Disease requiring supplemental oxygen was reported in less than 3% cases, and <1% were to be critically ill [1]. Therefore, understanding disease process and having a diagnosis are critical pieces of understanding. A group of findings that is particularly worrisome are cutaneous findings, and painful red and purple papules on fingers and toes have been colloquially termed

---

Editor Note: While at the current time (2023) COVID-19 has reached a global endemic state, its after effects are still being studied, and its impact on longitudinal pediatric growth is not fully understood.

S. Thikkurissy (✉)
Cincinnati Children's Hospital, Cincinnati, OH, USA
e-mail: Sarat.thikkurissy@cchmc.org

S. Thikkurissy, S. Golkari (eds.), *History and Physical for the Pediatric Dental Patient*, https://doi.org/10.1007/978-3-031-51458-6_12

"COVID toes" and as the differential can included coagulopathies should be referred and treated emergently [2].

A valuable tool in the pediatric dentist's armamentarium is the use of a directed history and physical (D-H&P). While the assessment of a child's overall health status may be straightforward in most cases, the child with a COVID-19 history may present some diagnostic challenges. These can be related to age of infection, symptomology, and subsequent need for supportive care (including supplemental oxygen). Therefore, dentists utilizing procedural sedation on pediatric patients should direct a physician comfortable with assessment of respiratory effort and post-viral assessment to evaluate the child's ability to tolerate treatment with sedatives (some of which may depress respiratory function/effort). The reason that a physician must be familiar with and comfortable with COVID symptoms and respiratory health is that there are specific diagnostic findings the physician should be aware of. On a typical complete blood count (CBC) with differential, there is slightly reduced white blood cell count, while progressive lymphocytopenia has been reported in more advanced cases. This reduction in lymphocytes when coupled with an increased creatine kinase may be suggestive of a more advanced form of COVID.

One of the most insidious and concerning outcomes in pediatric COVID-19 infection is multisystem inflammatory syndrome in children (MIS-C). According to Mehra et al., MIS-C is described as a "post-infectious, immune-mediated complication occurring 2 to 6 weeks after primary exposure, rather than an acute infection" [3]. This involves a severe neurologic insult that involves both the central and peripheral nervous system. The generally reported median age for MIS-C is 10 years old [4]. Roe continues to note that the "hyperinflammation (of MIS-C) coincides with peak antibody production several weeks after infection." [4] A concerning aspect of MIS-C is that, as per Belay, in a large US study of 1733 MIS-C patients, MIS-C primarily occurs after asymptomatic or relatively mild cases of COVID-19, and MIS-C does not occur during or after relatively severe cases of COVID-19. Additionally, these patients presented with higher levels of SARS-CoV-2 antibodies compared to peers [5]. Roe theorizes that the reason that children are predominantly targeted (and a small percentage at that) is related to the novel status of COVID-19 as an antigen. An accelerated production of antigen-antibody immune complexes occurs. This is paired with rare defects in complement, liver, and splenic immune responses leading to a Type III hypersensitivity reaction that is widespread.

Relating MIS-C to procedural sedation, assessment of residual pulmonary limitations post-COVID infection is critical. Furthermore, any unexplained rashes or dermatologic plaques should be referred for physician evaluation prior to proceeding with any sedation. A 2021 systematic review assessing over 3500 pediatric patients reported that 67% had abnormal chest CT findings, with 38% having bilateral lung involvement. The radiographic abnormalities included ground glass opacity (55%) and lung consolidation (10%) [6]. Saynhalath et al. concluded in their retrospective cohort study that "pediatric patients with non-severe SARS-CoV-2 infection had higher rates of peri anesthetic respiratory complications than matched controls with negative testing. However, severe morbidity was rare and there were no mortalities. The incidence of complications was similar to previously published rates of peri anesthetic complications in the setting of an upper respiratory tract infection" [7]. Traditionally, recommendations are that any nonemergent anesthetic/sedation be delayed 6 weeks post-resolution to allow for full recovery of airway from infection. Currently, there is a dearth of literature exploring specific procedural sedation outcomes in patients with a history of asymptomatic COVID-19 infection.

Another consideration the dentist must make is establishing the "true asymptomatic" nature of the COVID-19 infection. Some pediatric cases that are labeled "asymptomatic" may have indeed had elevation of temperature, nasal drainage, slight wheeze, or muscle pain. These may have not been recognized by parents due to unpredictable reporting ability of children, particularly preverbal children.

The American Society of Anesthesiologists in conjunction with the Anesthesia Patient Safety Foundation have released a joint statement on "Elective Surgery and Anesthesia for Patients after COVID-19 Infection." This statement terms "mild to moderate symptoms" as those not including viral pneumonia or oxygen saturation <94%. When examining a postinfection wait time, the document states "A multi-country (116 countries), multi-center (1674 hospitals) study of more than 140,000 patients, with 3,127 having COVID-19 infection before surgery, suggested that when possible, surgery should be delayed for at least 7 weeks following SARS-CoV-2 infection and that patients with ongoing symptoms at ≥7 weeks from diagnosis may benefit from further delay" [8].

The ASA document outlines suggested wait times from the date of COVID-19 diagnosis to surgery as follows [9]:

- Four weeks for an asymptomatic patient or recovery from only mild, non-respiratory symptoms.
- Six weeks for a symptomatic patient (e.g., cough, dyspnea) who did not require hospitalization.
- Eight to ten weeks for a symptomatic patient who is diabetic, immunocompromised, or hospitalized.
- Twelve weeks for a patient who was admitted to an intensive care unit due to COVID-19 infection.

Caution is *the* key word when electing to use procedural sedation on a pediatric patient who has a history of COVID-19 infection. The practitioner must balance the need for treatment, the ability to delay treatment (through such modalities as silver diamine fluoride and glass ionomer treatment), and the overall health status of the patient. Close consultation with a physician primary care is recommended, and as noted above, further in-depth consultation with pediatric pulmonary and/or infectious disease specialists may be of importance.

References

1. Alsohime F, Temsah M, Al-Nemri A, et al. COVID-19 infection prevalence in pediatric population: etiology, clinical presentation, and outcome. J Infect Public Health. 2020;13:1791–6.
2. Kolivras A, Dehavay F, Delplace D, et al. Coronavirus (COVID-19) infection induced chilblains: a case report with histopathologic findings. JAAD Case Rep. 2020;6(6):489–92. https://doi.org/10.1016/j.jdcr.2020.04.
3. Mehra B, Aggarwal Y, Dugaya S. MIS-C is a clinically different entity from acute COVID-19 in adults. Indian J Crit Care Med. 2021;25(8):954–5.
4. Roe K. Explanations for 10 of the most puzzling aspects of multisystem inflammatory syndrome and other Kawasaki-like diseases. J Clin Pharm Ther. 2021;47(4):539–43.
5. Belay ED, Abrams J, Oster ME, et al. Trends in geographical and temporal distribution of US children with multisystem inflammatory syndrome during the COVID-19 pandemic. JAMA Pediatr. 2021;175(8):837–45.
6. Ebrahimpour L, Marashi M, Zamanian H, et al. Computed tomography findings in 3,557 COVID-19 infected children: a systematic review. Quant Imaging Med Surg. 2021;11(11):4644–60.
7. Saynhalath R, Gijo A, Proshad E. Anesthetic complications associated with severe acute respiratory syndrome coronavirus 2 in pediatric patients. Anesth Analg. 2021;133(2):483–90.
8. Nepogodiev D, Simoes JFF, Li E, et al. Timing of surgery following SARS-CoV-2 infection: an international prospective cohort study. Anaesthesia. 2022;77(1):110.
9. APSF%20ASA%20Statement%20on%20Surgery%20after%20COVID%20rv%203-9-2021.pdf. Accessed 28 Oct 2021.